Oral Sex That'll Blow Her Mind

An Illustrated Guide to Giving Her Amazing Orgasms

Shanna Katz, M.Ed, ACS

Published by: AMORATA PRESS,
　　　　　　　an imprint of Ulysses Press
　　　　　　　P.O. Box 3440
　　　　　　　Berkeley, CA 94703
　　　　　　　www.amoratapress.com

ISBN13: 978-1-61243-028-7

Library of Congress Control Number: 2011913379

Printed in Korea by Tara TPS through Four Colour Imports

10 9 8 7 6 5 4 3 2 1

Acquisitions editor: Keith Riegert
Managing editor: Claire Chun
Editor: Paula Dragosh
Proofreader: Elyce Berrigan-Dunlop
Design and layout: Wade Nights
Production: Abigail Reser, Judith Metzener
Photographs: © Hollan Publishing, Inc.

Distributed by Publishers Group West

Contents

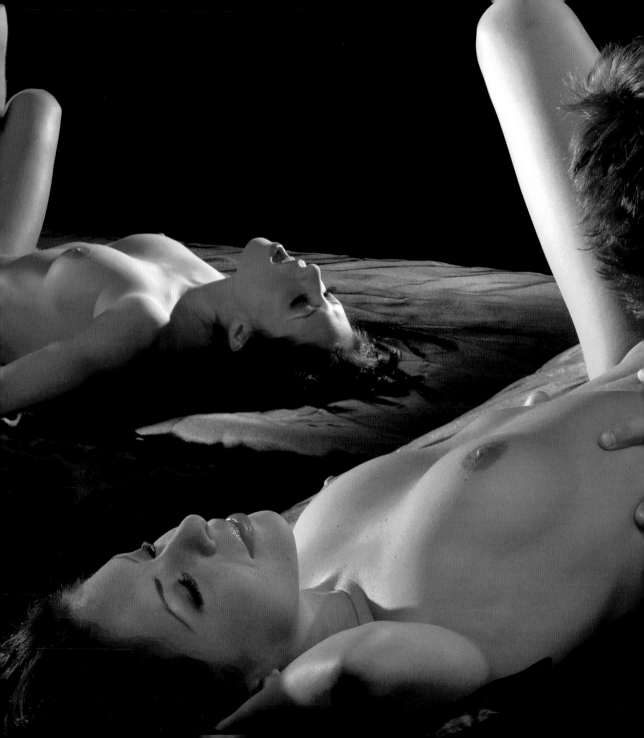

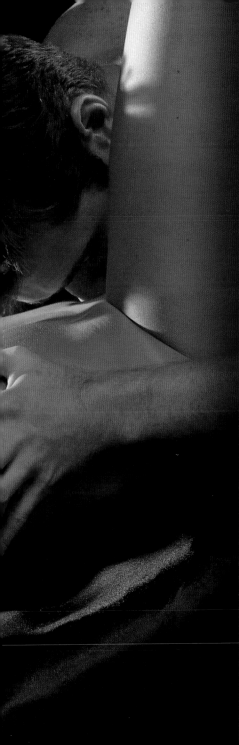

Introduction

✺ ✺ ✺

Of the many types of exciting sexual activities, which include massages, hand jobs, and all sorts of fabulous positions of intercourse, oral sex is a favorite of both couples and individuals. Depending on your partner, this could be fabulous fellatio, captivating cunnilingus, or admirable analingus.

But although many people like to fancy themselves as superstars in the bedroom, cunnilingus seems to be a frequent roadblock on the road to being number one in all things sex-tacular. Why? Lots of reasons! Many people have never even seen a vulva up close and personal (this includes lots of people WITH vulvas), and so pleasuring them can often seem like a mysterious act, something that perhaps takes a lifetime to master. There's also the question of timing, of what licks feel good versus which just fall flat and, of course, of how to know that your partner is truly enjoying your oral ministrations.

Lucky for you and other soon-to-be oral sex aficionados, this book has a whole lot of information in a little bit of space, so you can learn about basic vulvar anatomy, the ins and outs of smell and taste, and a bevy of tips and techniques in no time at all. Whether you're just

getting started in the wonderful world of oral sex or looking to improve your style, *Blow Her Mind* is here to help you be the leader of the lickers!

One of the most important aspects of healthy and enjoyable sex is the ability to communicate with your partner. Whether you're having a quick and dirty hookup in a bar bathroom or looking to spice things up with your life partner, communication is key, especially for sex and fun in the bedroom (or wherever you're up to naughtiness and sexy times). This book has some tips and techniques to improve your cunnilingus skills and to educate you on vulvar anatomy, but it also includes fun activities and ideas to increase communication and even intimacy in your partnerships. The more you

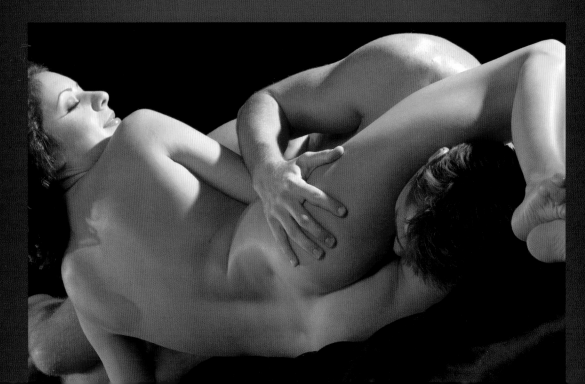

communicate, the more your wants and needs are expressed, the more you can understand the wants and needs of your partner, and the better the sex is overall.

So enjoy this book. You can read it from beginning to end, section by section, or stick your finger in, close your eyes, and just go with the flow (don't try this with a vulva—most vulvas appreciate a little direction and not so much guesswork). Take the parts that are relevant to you and your current or potential partners, and leave the rest. Should you need it in the future, the information will always be there.

What Is Cunnilingus?

There are lots of slang terms for cunnilingus, including going down, dining downtown, eating out, carpet munching, muff diving, dining at the Y, clam digging, having a box lunch (which is a true favorite!), and enjoying the breakfast of champions. Whatever you call it, cunnilingus is the oral (mouth) stimulation of the entire vulva (clitoris, labia, and vaginal opening).

The idea of getting naked and going down on someone can be nerve-racking for anyone. But once the tongue gets going, most people enjoy cunnilingus immensely, both the act of giving and, of course, receiving. Let's look at some of the reasons why!

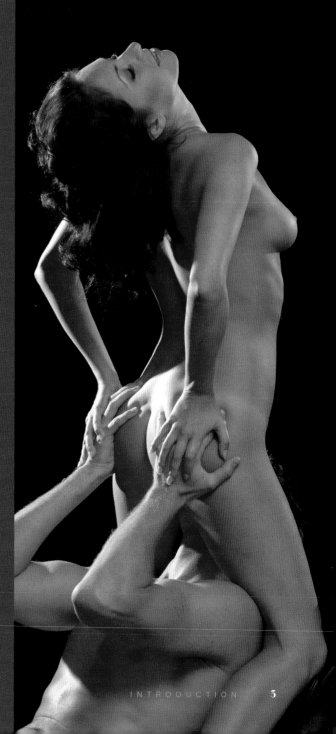

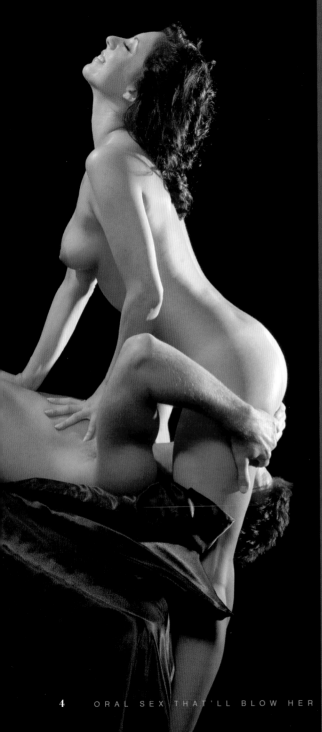

Why Many People Might Enjoy Receiving Cunnilingus

It can feel REALLY good—physically, sexually, and mentally.

Cunnilingus can be incredibly intimate for some people, helping them feel more grounded and connected with their partner.

For some people, cunnilingus is the only way that they can achieve orgasm with a partner.

For other people, cunnilingus before, during, or after other sexual activities can boost their libido and endorphins, making their experiences feel even better and sexier.

Some receivers find receiving cunnilingus to be a very sexy or powerful act.

Cunnilingus can provide a different sensation than fingers, a vibrator, intercourse, or other activities might. Each person likes different types of stimulation, and this might be the one that really gets their heart pounding.

The receiver of cunnilingus has significantly more control over the types and locations of sensations that they're receiving by moving their hips around to get the tongue to their sweet spot.

The person receiving cunnilingus can relax and focus on getting pleasure from their partner, rather than feel as if they need to be giving pleasure at the same time. This relaxation can

(text continued on p. 9)

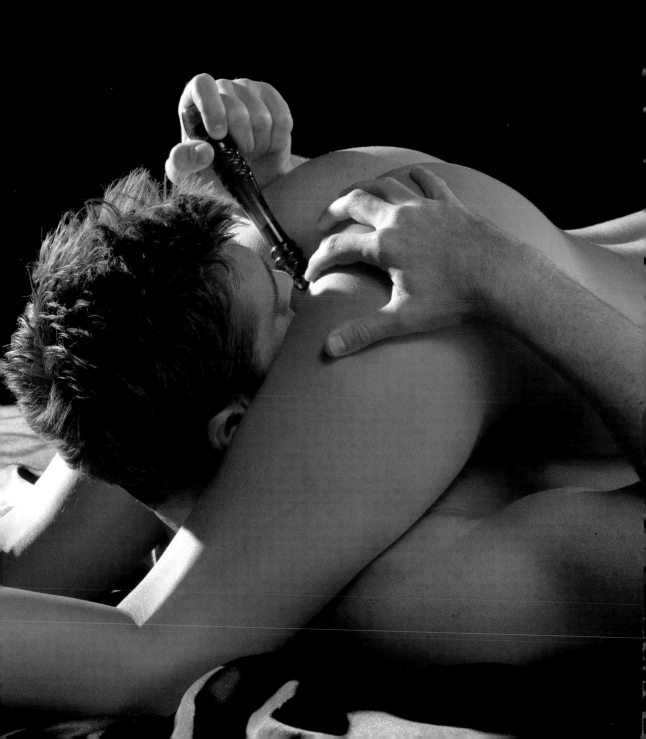

Cunnilingus Myths

Myth

Everyone can orgasm from cunnilingus — if they can't, something's wrong with them.

Busted

Hmmm. Usually statements about sex and orgasms like "Everyone can . . ." are bound to be false. Although many, many, many people can in fact orgasm from vulvar stimulation, not everyone can, and not everyone can every time that they receive cunnilingus. Bodies (everyone's bodies!) are constantly changing, and even if someone has had an orgasm from getting eaten out once, factors like stress, medication, different stages of the menstrual cycle, and so on could keep it from happening each and every time. Moreover, if someone doesn't reach orgasm from epic oral ministrations, that's absolutely fine, too. All that matters is that they're enjoying it and that it feels good!

If we look at sex from a more pleasure-based model, where success is everyone enjoying themselves and having a fabulous time, it takes pressure off everyone involved. The person receiving the cunnilingus can focus on all of the delicious sensations rather than feel as if they must reach this socially created orgasmic place, and the person providing the oral sex can focus on providing pleasure to their partner instead of heading toward some randomly described goal. If orgasm happens, then great . . . but if they don't, it doesn't mean that anyone's failed. Remember, with sex, fun should be the name of the game!

Granted, not everyone likes receiving oral sex. Some people find the stimulation too light for them, others prefer different activities, and some may have had a bad experience with a previous partner. It's also possible that someone's dislike of oral sex may be culturally based. If you're set on going downtown, and your partner isn't into it, you can ask why. Maybe they're worried about the way they taste, and that can be an easy fix (see Myth TK). But if they don't want you to go down on them, they don't want it, and it's absolutely not OK to argue with or convince them otherwise. Take all of that fabulous sexual pleasure energy and work on creating a pleasurable situation as part of a different sexual activity! Figure out what other kind of sexual interaction you both enjoy, and work on getting pleasure to happen that way.

Myth

Every woman loves getting cunnilingus for hours.

Busted

Everyone's sexual preferences are different. Some people LOVE receiving oral and are as happy as a clam (pun intended) for hours on end while their nether regions are getting some lip service. Others like oral sex as part of an evening of activities, before or after another type of sexual adventure. And others don't like receiving oral at all, in any way, shape, or form. So what's the best way to figure out what your partner wants in regard to oral? Ask! Communication is key, and it's a surefire way to give your partner the best possible pleasure, based on what they like and don't like, want and don't want.

You may want to bring up bad experiences with sex, whether it's receiving cunnilingus or sexual interaction in general. Some people may have had a partner they didn't trust or something that just physically didn't feel good. They might be a survivor of sexual coercion or assault. If so, letting them talk about their wants, needs, concerns, and limits is a great way to figure out where they are on receiving cunnilingus. It's possible that they might be interested in having you go down on them, but are unsure how to ask for it, how they might react, or how they might feel if they do enjoy it.

Getting these concerns out in the open allows you both to come up with plans for any and all possible outcomes, and for you to reassure your partner of your caring and support. It's also possible that they're just not down with you going down, for whatever reason. As I said above, it's never OK to be pushy. It's OK to ask why; it's not OK to keep bugging them about it. There's a whole world out there of sexual things that are fun and enjoyable; find the ones that you both like, and start going at it like bunnies!

Myth

If I do exactly what I see in porn, my partner will orgasm like a rocket.

Busted

If you're one of the millions of folks who enjoys porn, remember, it's not usually an accurate reflection of reality. Much of pornography is about fulfilling fantasies, and for many people, that means women on-screen who are turned on by everything and can orgasm at the slightest touch, and men on-screen who are sexual rock stars, always erect with larger than average penises. If you enjoy watching that on-screen, that's 100 percent fine. But it's important to remember that a bedroom and a porn set are completely different. You don't get to see what happens between takes, such as who's masturbating to lead to more arousal, who's adding lube or giving their vibrator a little action, and how much of each scene ends up on the cutting floor. Even if an orgasm from cunnilingus is authentic, you have no idea what led up to it—you see only what the director and producers want you to see.

Are some people exactly like folks in porn? Probably. But the majority of sexually active adults don't look like most porn stars, and their sex lives don't follow a script; most people's sexual activities tend to be just as varied as the genres of mainstream pornography. People tend to want a little bit more time at each stage, tend to want to switch positions less often, and need a lot more stimulation for sex to be pleasurable. This isn't a reason to stop watching porn, but it's a reason to look at the reality of sex with your partner and figure out what will make sex the most enjoyable for the two of you, rather than trying to re-create what you saw on the screen.

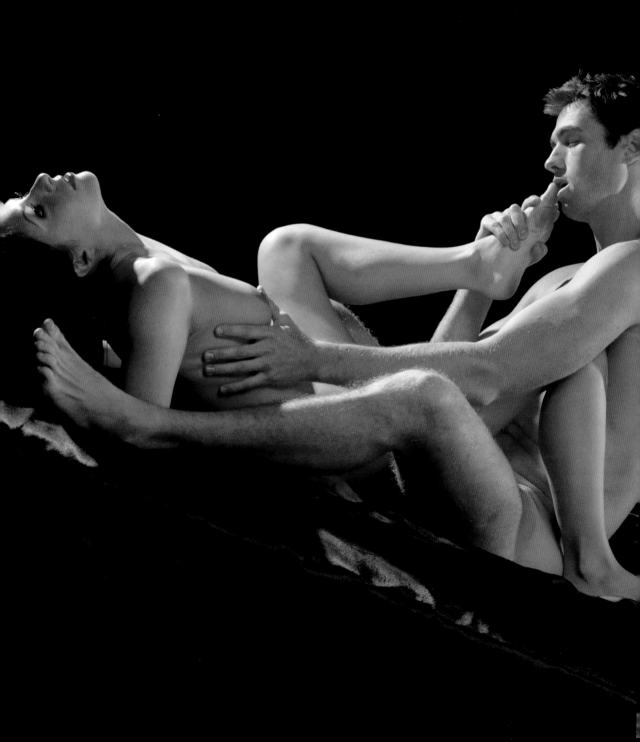

help many folks reach orgasm if stress was a roadblock before.

Why Many People Might Enjoy Giving Cunnilingus

It feels REALLY good to give your partner pleasure, and since so many people enjoy receiving cunnilingus, this is an easy way to provide direct pleasure to the person you're with.

Cunnilingus can be incredibly intimate for some people, helping them feel more grounded and connected with their partner, whether they're the giver or the receiver.

The giver can focus on giving pleasure and not be worried about their own orgasm, erection, lubrication. All they need to do is focus on their partner.

The offering of cunnilingus can be used as part of power play, either as a reward or as a nice, long, drawn-out tease to get someone really turned on.

Most people love helping their partner orgasm, and cunnilingus is a great way to do this. While not everyone loves cunnilingus or can achieve orgasm from it, many people find it to be the best way for them to orgasm or to get them turned on for other sexual adventures.

Cunnilingus can be a great way to relax your body while providing pleasure to your partner.

So with all of these absolutely fabulous reasons to give and get cunnilingus, why the heck would anyone not be lined up for dinner at the Y?

With the caveat that some people just plain don't like receiving oral sex, and that's 100 percent OK—to each their own—let's talk about some reasons that cunnilingus may seem mysterious, difficult, or even weird to some people.

First, there are a lot of myths around the vagina, the vulva, and cunnilingus. I'll be talking about the anatomy of the vulva a little bit later, but for now, let's get started with some myth busting.

A Note on Gender: The spectrum of sexuality is huge and rarely discussed. A variety of gender identities encompass people as a whole. Not all women-identified people have a vulva, and not everyone with a vulva identifies as a woman. Throughout this book, I'll be using the term woman and the pronouns she, her, and hers for ease of reading. But it's important to keep in mind that anyone with a vulva can enjoy cunnilingus and that not everyone with a vulva uses feminine pronouns.

A Note on Orientation: ANYONE, regardless of gender, sex, or orientation, can provide outstanding cunnilingus. This book has been written using the word partner (rather than girlfriend/boyfriend or husband/wife) and nongendered pronouns to allow for the diversity of relationships and the fact that anyone can be a fabulous muff diver.

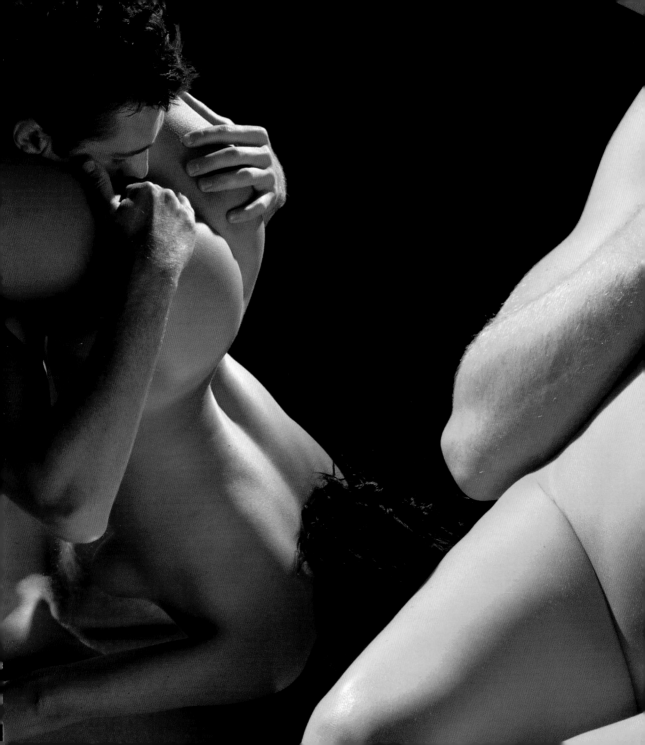

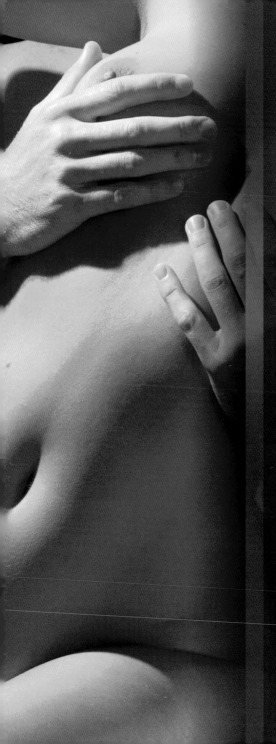

Anatomy

* * *

OK, so why am I using the term vulva instead of vagina?

While the vagina is part of the vulva, the vulva is not part of the vagina.

As you can see, the vulva is the whole enchilada: the mons pubis, both inner and outer labia, the clitoris, the clitoral hood, the urethra, and the vagina (plus the perineum at the base of all this). Unfortunately, because we don't talk about our genitals, especially these genitals, many people are a bit uninformed as to what the difference is between the vulva and the vagina. Sit down, and prepare to absorb some sexy anatomy information coming at ya!

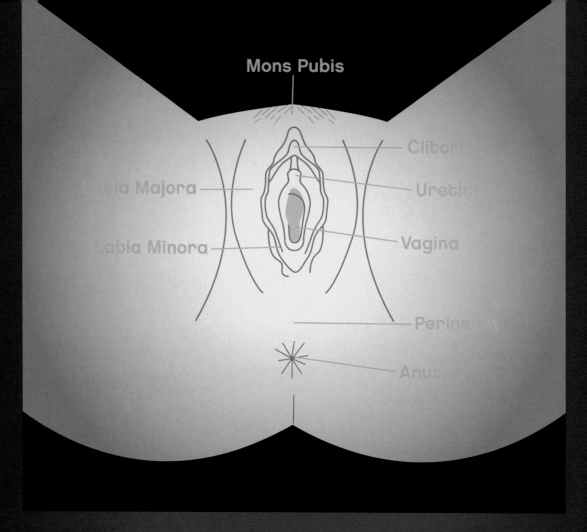

Mons Pubis

Clitoris

Urethra

Labia Majora

Vagina

Labia Minora

Perineum

Anus

People have all sorts of interesting names for this area, including pussy, punani, vag, vajay-jay, puss, little man in the canoe, special place, labbe, cooter, cunt, yoni, snatch, po-po, junk, coochie, flower, cave of wonders, petals, breakfast of champions, lady bits, baby maker, business, snapper, pink taco, clam, schmende, beaver, box, mimi, tottita, tamale, and more!

Mons Pubis

The mons pubis is often referred to as the pubic bone, or the Mound of Venus, depending on who's talking. It, like the labia major/outer labia, is naturally covered in pubic hair (although some people choose to trim/shave/decorate this hair). It can be fun to rub, touch, and stroke this area. Because the nerves of the clitoris actually extend under this area, many people like to have it pressed on with the palm of the hand, either their own or their partner's. It can be a great area to begin stimulation before you dive in for the main course of cunnilingus.

Labia

As for the labia, the Latin gets it a little wrong. According to the scientific terms, these lips are known as the labia majora (big lips) and labia minora (little lips). But this is often incorrect. Vulvas are like snowflakes: each one is completely different. Sometimes the labia minora are larger than the labia majora, sometimes they're the same size, sometimes they are smaller, and sometimes labia on the same vulva can be different sizes — it's all perfectly normal. So I'm going to stick with calling them the inner lips and the outer lips, as those are never reversed.

The outer lips also come naturally graced with pubic hair (again, whether or not people choose to keep that hair is entirely up to them) and lie on either side of the vulva, oftentimes enclosing everything else. The inner lips are thinner, hairless, and can either be tucked between the outer lips or extend beyond them. It's completely normal for the lips to be uneven, to have different coloration, and so forth. Nothing that a person does (short of surgery, which is strongly NOT recommended unless health issues are at play) can change the size or length of the inner

labia. Their appearance is in no way correlated with how many people they have had sex with, the age at which they started having sex, the size of the toys/hands/penises they put inside them, and so forth. Whatever size, shape, color, and length that these inner lips are is exactly the way that they're supposed to be, period.

Most people like having their labia stimulated and played with. Some will enjoy gentle stroking and a soft touch, others want a little bit of pulling, or maybe some nibbling. And some like it rough. The easiest way to figure out what you like is to experiment a little, and assuming that your partner has a vulva (or that you're interested in playing with a vulva at some point), just ASK them how they like their lips to be touched. Communication is always the best way to figure out how touch feels for someone else, including what feels good and what does NOT feel good.

Clitoris

The inner lips lead up to the top of the vulva, forming the clitoral hood, which is a cover for the actual clitoris itself. This hood is a thin covering of skin that protects the very sensitive clitoris from too much stimulation before it's ready, and can also be enjoyable to touch as well. It acts almost as an eyelid, covering up the clit from the outside world. This covering is important, because without it, the clitoris would be rubbed and stimulated all day long, simply from walking, sitting and standing, riding a bike, and so forth. While that might sound like paradise to some, it could certainly get old and not feel so good after a while.

Now, most people think the clitoris is just the glans below the clitoral hood. Not true! In fact, the clitoris is shaped similarly to a wishbone and has long legs that extend down below the vulva, underneath the labia (one reason why it feels so good to stimulate the labia as well as the clitoral glans). The clitoris is just packed full of amazing-feeling nerve endings and has no other purpose in the human body than to create pleasure. How fabulous is that?

As a person gets more aroused, the clitoral hood will pull back slightly, allowing more access to the clitoral glans. Sometimes, when a person is close to orgasm, the hood will once again cover the glans, which can be incredibly frustrating. It's OK if this happens—just keep on stimulating or licking, and remember that this means that you're right on target. The hood and the glans love being touched (especially with lube—check out the section on lubricants to choose one that's friendly for vulvas), although not always directly. Many people also like oral stimulation of the lips, hood, and clitoris, whether it's licking, sucking, or gentle nibbling. Other vulva owners enjoy the feeling of vibrators on their clitoris, providing a different type of stimulation than fingers can. Each to their own!

Urethra

Between the clitoral glans/hood and vaginal opening is the urethra, which is where urine comes out. For those people who can ejaculate during G-spot stimulation, this is where the ejaculatory fluid comes out. Keep in mind that ejaculatory fluid from vulvas is NOT urine—it's produced in the skein's gland and has a different composition than urine. It's completely normal to experience vulvar ejaculation, and equally normal not to. It's fun to experiment, but not being able to ejaculate doesn't mean anything negative. The same is true vice versa; being able to ejaculate doesn't mean anything is wrong with you. Either way, ejaculation is not the holy grail of sexual play. Some people love it, and other people wish they didn't have to wash their towel quite as often because of their ejaculatory loving.

Many people enjoy have the area around the urethra (the urinary meatus) stimulated gently with a finger, although few people actually want any penetration of this area. Always be gentle, and stimulate this area only with clean fingers or clean toys. Getting foreign bacteria up the urethra is just asking for a urinary tract infection, and that's absolutely no fun.

Vagina

Now we've made it to the vagina! Can you see how many other parts of the vulva there are, and how much lovely stimulation one can get from

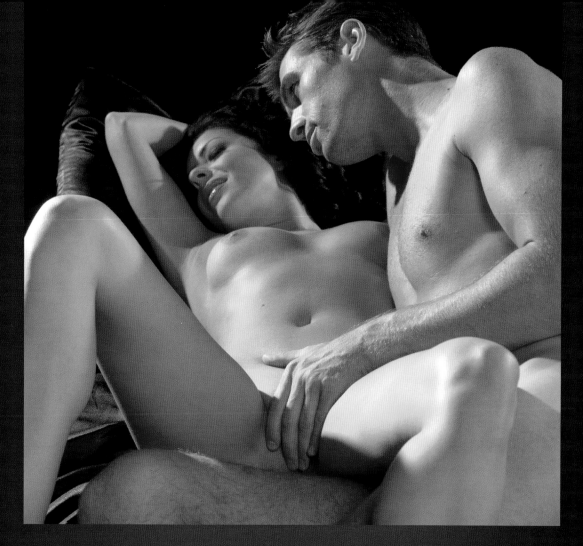

them? True, the vagina is pretty awesome, but so is the rest of the vulva. Also, while the vagina is great and all that, it doesn't usually play a starring role in the actual act of cunnilingus. Contrary to popular belief, unless your tongue is as long as Gene Simmons's (or longer), most human tongues cannot reach too far into the vagina. Most of the stimulation you'll be giving when you're dining at the Y will be all around the vulva. Only if your partner likes internal stimulation while receiving oral (from lubed fingers or toys) does the vagina actually come into play.

Vulvar Viewing Party

Part of learning to love the vulva, the vagina, and the whole enchilada is taking some time to get to know it. Can you hop into bed, undress, and go muff diving without a second thought? Absolutely. But some of the best cunnilingus connoisseurs also take more time to get to know each and every individual vulva. How can you get in on this appreciation of the cave of wonders?

Step 1

Make sure there's proper lighting. Some people may have concerns about getting down with the lights on. If your partner isn't in love with the idea of fluorescent bulbs beating down on them, you have plenty of alternatives. Bathe the room in romantic candlelight, or go exploring under the covers with a flashlight. However you choose to light your space, get some rays on the vulva in front of you before you begin your moment of appreciation.

Step 2

Make sure you have time. If you're just getting down for a quickie, this is probably not the right time to sit down and learn to truly love the vulva in front of you. Ditto if you have friends or folks coming over, or water boiling on the stove. Wait until you have a good bit of time to really learn and explore this beautiful breakfast of champions you behold before you.

Step 3

Help the vulva owner to relax and enjoy the experience. To be honest, most people have never had a partner sit them down and tell them that they want to check them out . . . down below. Our culture is so fixated with the actual acts of sex that most of the time, we don't get to stop and smell the roses, if you know what I mean. Exploring your partner's petals may make them a little nervous or apprehensive that you might not like what you see: reassure them that you're excited to get your own personal viewing of their vivacious vulva, as well as to get to know all the ins and outs of their naughty bits to provide them with more pleasure. Once you both relax and get into it, it can be a great experience.

Step 4

Provide positive feedback. Every single one of us is nervous about our bodies in some way, and that anxiety can intensify when it comes to our genitals. When you've placed yourself between your partner's legs, it's the time to let them know your full appreciation. Whether you're the type to oooh and ahhh, or you're more the type to provide a play-by-play ("Wow — that's the most gorgeous set of labia I've ever seen! Now I'm going to check out your sexy clitoral hood before I delve deeper!"), make sure that you're providing constant and positive feedback. We all want to hear about how much others are turned on by us, and now is definitely a time to share it.

Step 5

Take it all in. If your partner has pubic hair, run your finger through it. If you like the smell of vulvas, or perhaps have never smelled one before, take a good whiff, as each and every vulva has a unique scent. Feel the different labia between your fingers. Really explore the vulva in front of you, and more importantly, make mental notes. Always begin gently, and feel free to use lube. Note what makes your partner squirm in a good way, and what seems to be a no-fly zone.

Step 6

Put your knowledge to use. After your careful and exciting explorations and examinations, take what you've learned and use it in the field. While it's nice to look and touch, it can be even nicer to use your newfound information while actually playing with the vulva and performing cunnilingus. Perhaps you've discovered a special zone that gets your partner going, or you've learned that they get incredibly turned on when you run your fingers across their mons. Whatever information you garnered during your exploratory time, now is the time to make it work for you. Go forth, experiment, and enjoy!

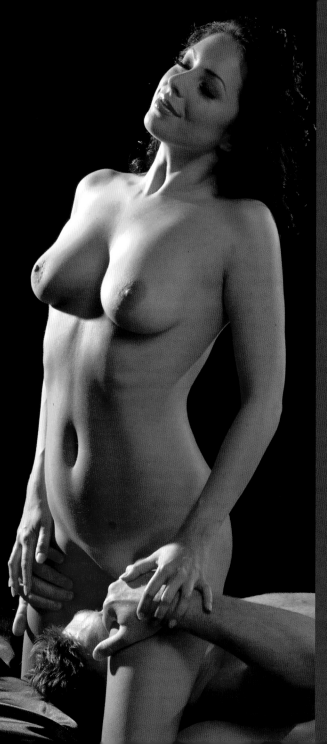

The vaginal opening is pretty self-explanatory—it's the opening to the vagina, jam-packed with fabulous nerves. Lots of people like having the opening gently stroked and played with, regardless of whether anything will be going inside. Keep in mind that while many vulvas naturally lubricate, some don't, and extra lube is almost always welcome. Having some extra lube handy (that's vulva friendly) can earn you an extra A+ on your vulva-loving report card.

Just past the vaginal opening is the vaginal canal, what most people refer to as the vagina. Vaginas vary in depth; the average is five to eight inches. But some can be shallower, especially if there's an inverted uterus. The majority of the sensation is in the front third of the vagina, which is why many people say that they prefer girth more so than length in their partners and/ or toys. It's also why a lot of folks report that they like the first few strokes of being penetrated (whether by fingers, toys, or penises), because they tend to be the shallowest, and they really stimulate this area. As discussed above, the legs of the clitoris run under the labia and actually hug the opening of the vaginal canal, helping provide these delicious-feeling sensations.

Cervix

At the end of the vaginal canal is the cervix, with a tiny opening called the os. The cervix is like a cap on the end of the vagina — nothing can go farther. The os will open slightly to allow out menstrual fluid and may dilate to allow a baby through during birth, but otherwise it's closed. This means that you CANNOT lose things in the vagina — not toys, not tampons, not fingers. It's a closed system, some might say.

As for stimulation of the cervix, this is another one of those love-hate dichotomies, and it's important to know your partner's preferences before you start rubbing or poking the cervix. For some people, this can feel incredibly good, like a supersensual internal massage. For others, simply touching the cervix can lead to epic cramping, and with that, there is no possibility for any more sex. Talk to your partner; they might not know, but if they do, you can sure save yourself a world of trouble later on!

PC/Kegel Muscles

Want to experience deeper, stronger, and more intense vaginal orgasms? All you have to do is work out!

Squeeze your muscles in as if you're trying to stop the flow of your urine (you CAN try it while peeing to help find your muscles, but please don't try to stop the flow of your pee often — it's not good for your body). Then push out. Squeeze in. And again. Those are your PC/kegel muscles. To work them out, you can squeeze in and hold for five to ten seconds and let out, or pulse them in and out for thirty seconds, or create any routine you want. Just like any other muscle group, you have to start slowly and build up to more repetitions. After working your muscles out a while, you can hold them in for a longer period. It can also be fun to do these exercises while you have a hand/penis/toy inside you. If you need a little extra help, try kegel balls (meant to be worn while you walk around, to help you with your exercises), kegelcisors, or kegel barbells.

If you're not the owner of the vulva in question, don't worry; you can enjoy the excitement of exercising the PC/kegel muscles as well. Gently slide a lubed finger or two into your partner (after reading the section on lubricants and which ones are vulva friendly), and once your partner's warmed up and used to you, have them squeeze their muscles as described above. You should be able to feel the walls of their vagina clamping down on you, and then letting up. Have them do different patterns, squeezing for different amounts of time. And because everyone can work out their PC muscles regardless of their genitalia, both of you can work out your PC muscles at the same time. Finally, a type of exercise that EVERYONE can have fun doing!

G-spot

Now that we've gotten the excitement of the PC muscles and kegel exercises out of the way, that brings us to the G-spot, sometimes called the urethral sponge. Named after the original discoverer/proponent, Dr. Grafenberg, the Grafenberg spot (a.k.a. G-spot) is about one to three inches inside the vaginal canal, at the top, and it usually feels kind of spongy or bumpy, almost like the roof of your mouth. It can usually be found either with a toy that has a nice curve or by inserting fingers into the vagina and making a "come here" motion.

The important thing to note about the G-spot (well, one of many!) is that it doesn't always exist. No, it's true! In fact, the G-spot exists only when the G-spot owner is incredibly aroused. This has made it difficult for many scientific studies of the G-spot to be done, given that most folks are not incredibly turned on by having their feet in stirrups in the gynecologist's office. But many, many, many studies have been done, and have been accepted by various scientific communities, that prove the existence of this area and that it can cause pleasure in some folks. Just like any other part of the body, the G-spot will feel different to different people and people may like to have this area stimulated in different ways. While for some people, stimulating the G-spot is akin to finding the holy grail, others may find it to be just "meh" or even annoying. As usual, ask your partner for their feelings on it!

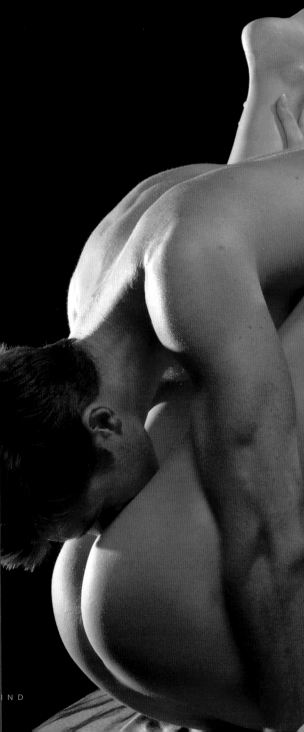

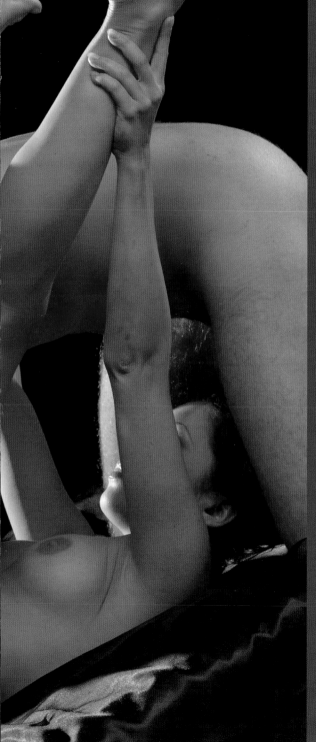

Perineum and Anus

At the end of all of this vulvar goodness lies the perineum. Everyone has one of these! For some bodies, it's between the base of the scrotum and the anus . . . for others, it's between the vaginal opening and the anus. Some people call this the "'tain't" (it 'tain't the balls/vagina, and it 'tain't the ass), others call it a pleasure zone, and more names abound. This area is filled with more nerve endings, and a lot of people find it to be very pleasurable when it's stimulated.

At the far side of the perineum is the anus. Now, the anus is not actually part of the vulva, and it contains all of its own nerves and fun tricks. But some people like to pair anal action with their receiving of cunnilingus, so it's important to bring it up. The anus is not naturally dirty, and you certainly don't need an enema or douche to clean it up. If you're concerned, put a bit of warm water in a blue squeezy syringe from the drugstore and rinse it out. Because anal tissue is incredibly delicate, you want to make sure that you're always careful and gentle when playing with this area, both externally and internally. Also, the anus provides no natural lubricant. This means that it's absolutely crucial to add lube when playing with the back door. Check out the section on lubricant to learn more about the different varieties of lube available for use.

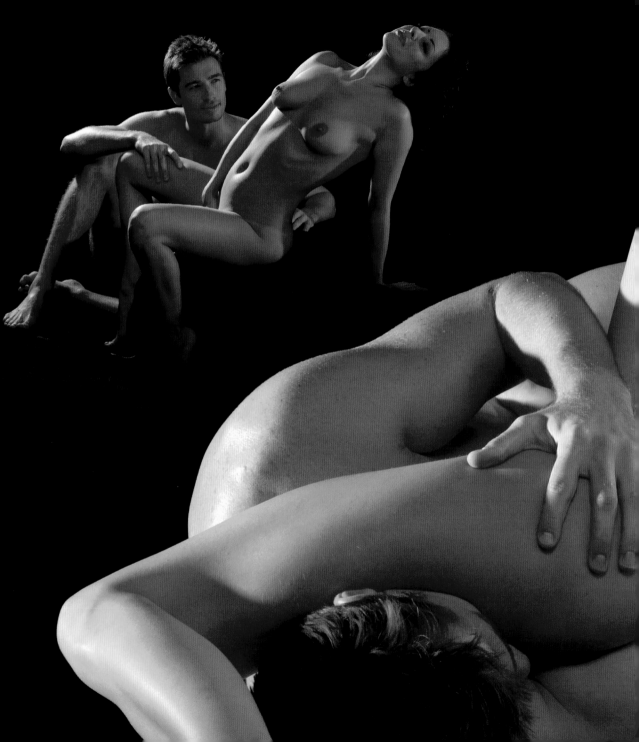

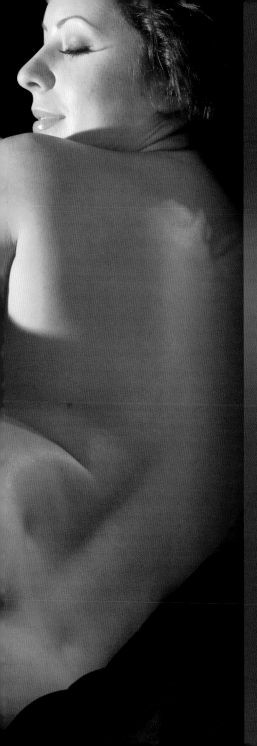

Communication

If you read this book and put it down with only one take-home message, let it be Communication Is Key. Vulvas (and humans, for that matter) were not built One Size Fits All, and they certainly don't come with downloadable manuals for owners or their partners. Many people with vulvas are still in the midst of trying to figure out what their own vulva likes and doesn't like, what its needs are, and how to communicate them. Sometimes, they like something one day, and something different the next. Sometimes more feels good, and other times, less is much, much, much more. The best way to be an amazing partner in the sack is to communicate. This

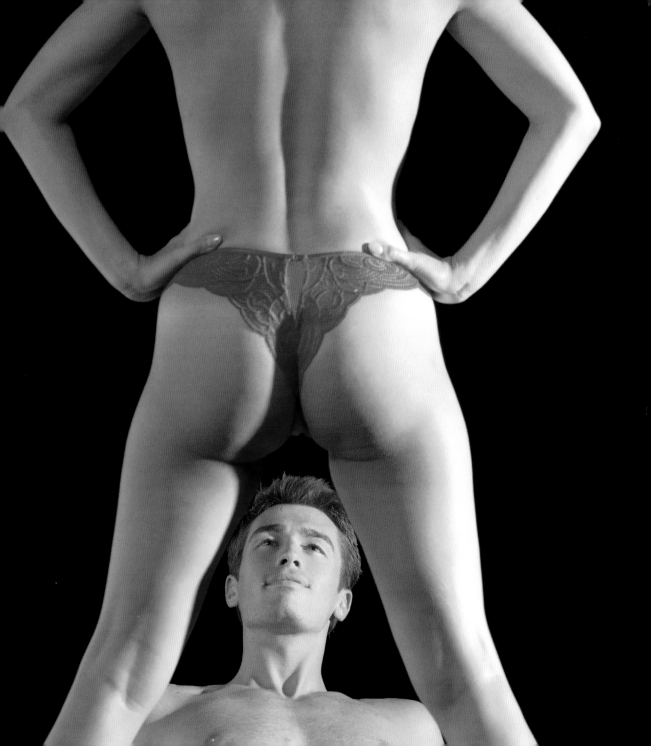

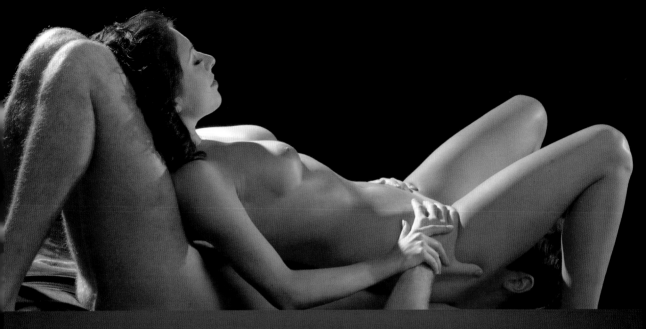

means not only sharing your own wants and needs but also asking for feedback from your partner. The kicker is that when you ask for feedback, you have to not only listen but also assimilate said feedback into your lovemaking, fucking, or knocking off socks.

Communication doesn't always have to be verbal. Figure out which types of communication work best for you and which types work best for your partner. It's possible that one of you needs the most direct communication possible: "Lick me lightly at this exact location for this amount of time before switching to a more intense direct licking at this location until I say to move." It's equally possible that one of you might prefer certain levels of moaning, or pulling of the hair, or placing your partner's hand on top of your own to guide you to the right

areas and amounts of pressure. Text messages can be sexy communication throughout the day or week: "Love it when u lick me with ur finger inside me" or "Tease me 4ever before u finally touch me" can provide lots of direction for the pleasure giver. Even sitting together to watch porn or read erotica can be a great way of saying "Oooh—I really like that! Maybe you could try it on me" or "Wow, that position looks really uncomfortable; I wonder how we could get that angle without me breaking my neck?"

Here are some exercises to help you with sexual communication with your partner. Try some of them out and see if they apply to you and your relationship. If they work, then congrats. Use your newfound communication skills often. If they don't work for you, try different ones, or experiment with your own!

Compliment Sandwich

This is where you provide feedback to your partner in a sandwich of the following:

Positive Comment

Suggestion for Change

Positive Comment

See, it's a sandwich where the two slices of bread are fabulous (and genuine) compliments. These help remind your partner of how much you enjoy being with them, and enjoy being sexual with them, while also providing you with the opportunity to ask for any change that you may be wanting. Here are two examples.

Example #1

Wow — you look so fucking sexy with your head between my legs!

I wish you could spend more time down there . . .

It really turns me on when you go down on me!

Example #2

You're so incredibly sexy with your hot moaning . . .

I'd love it if you'd pull my hair when something feels really good!

It's really hot for me to get to eat you out!

The middle layer can be feedback about timing, positions, pressure, noise (or lack thereof), and so forth. Whatever you need to communicate to your partner (regardless of whether you're the cunnilingus giver or receiver), you can try out a compliment sandwich to get the message across while still validating your partner's sexiness and sexual prowess.

The "Let Me Show You" Approach

Every vulva will have different pleasure spots and desired pressure at different times. Sometimes, this'll correlate with the menstrual cycle, and other times, this may come at random. It's a fact of sex. One great way to figure out what the vulva in front of you wants is to ask its owner to show you. Place a lubed finger or hand on the vulva, and have the owner (yourself or your partner) place one of their hands/fingers on top of yours. Let them guide your hand or finger around their vulva, slowly at first, showing you which areas feel good and demonstrating the amount of pressure that feels best to them by pressing down on your hand or finger. As they get going, they can speed up the movement, or they can slow it down, move around the vulva, and so forth, to demonstrate exactly the areas, speeds, and pressures that feel best to them. After this, show them that you're a star pupil, and show off what you've just learned.

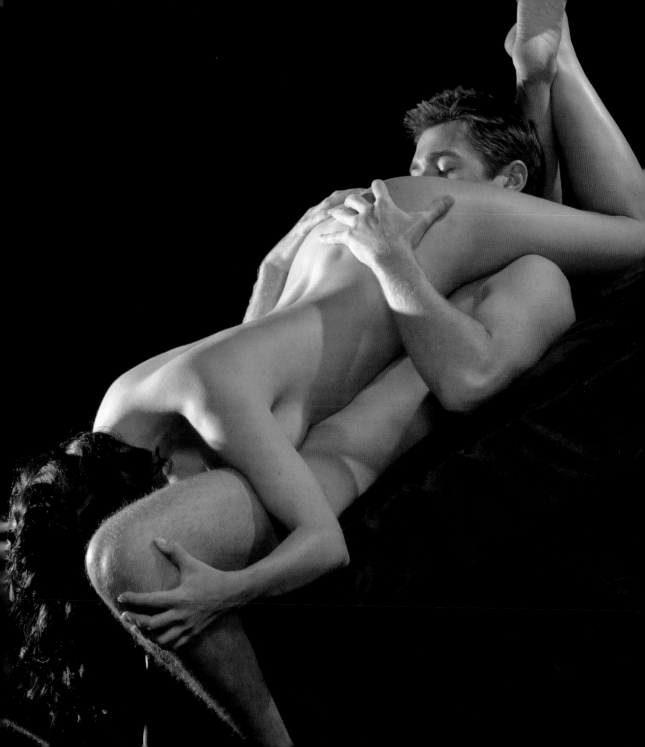

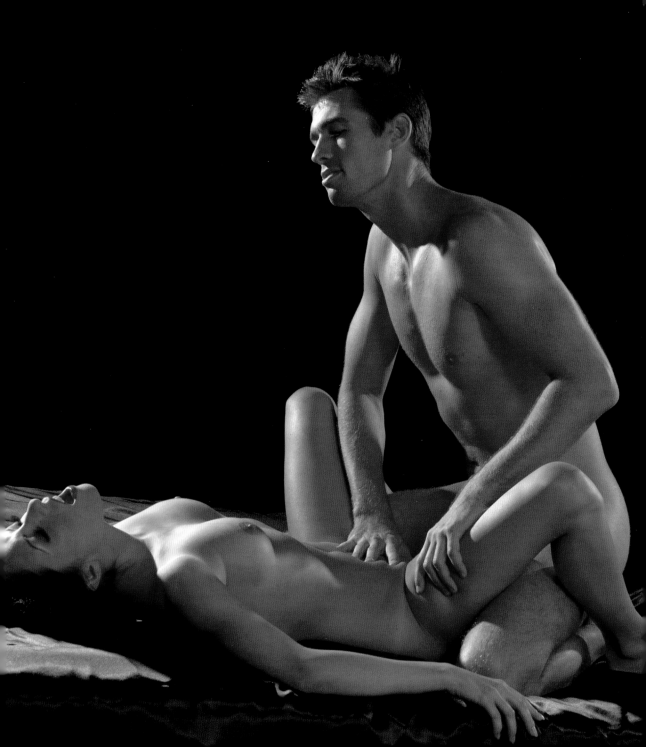

The Secret Code

You can, with the help of your partner, create a code of sorts to let the giver of cunnilingus know how things are going. Perhaps the receiver will moan loudly for "Yes, yes!," groan quietly for "harder," and pant for "softer." Maybe it's the hair-pulling action as reins, where the receiver of cunnilingus will pull on the hair/head of the giver based on the sensation they'd like: left means left, right means right, pulling inward means more pressure, while pulling outward means less pressure. Whatever works best for the two of you, decide on a code and make sure you practice it . . . over and over.

Rock around the Clock

With the concept of looking between the cunnilingus receiver's legs at the vulva (with them on their back, and the cunnilingus giver on their front), picture the vulva as the face of a clock, with the top of the clitoral hood being twelve and the perineum (or right under the vagina) being six. The two of you can then, with a lubricated finger or adventurous tongue, rock your way around the clock to figure out which areas feel best when stimulated and what type of pressure feels best for each number. Many folks find that the two-three area is their favorite, although each person will certainly have a favorite number or even combination of numbers. This can lead to a

great synonym for oral, telling your partner that it's three o'clock and time to get down . . . if you know what I mean.

Show and Tell

While this isn't up every set of partners' alley, show and tell can be a great way for a person to learn about their partner's vulva, and what feels good. Have the person who's going to do the show and tell get comfortable (in bed, on a couch, wherever), and then begin to masturbate. This can include lube, fingers, toys, and more. Watch them, from start to whatever the end might look like. First, this can be an incredibly sexy experience, watching your partner take control of their own pleasure. It can also be an intimate experience for some people. Second, it gives the "voyeur" a better idea of what things feel good to their partner; perhaps they spent a lot of time on nipple stimulation before reaching below the belt. Maybe they used a lot of insertion, or maybe none at all. Possibly, lube played a bigger role than one might think, or maybe there was just barely a hint of touch. Whatever it looks like, one partner gets to put on a fabulous show, and the other partner gets to enjoy the show while learning a lot. A win-win situation.

Vagina Myths

Myth

Vaginas and vulvas smell bad/taste bad.

Busted

Vaginas and vulvas smell and taste the way that they're SUPPOSED to smell and taste. Everyone has a unique scent and taste, and some people can even pick out their partner while blindfolded, just from smelling or tasting them. Pretty cool, right?

Now, if there's a fishy smell, that can indicate bacterial vaginosis (a bacterial infection that can be easily treated by a doctor) and should be looked at by a gynecologist.

But for the most part, vaginal odor is natural, usually a little musky, and similar to the muskiness of the penis/testicles. As long as your partner practices good hygiene and bathes regularly, you're good to go.

Still worried about it, either about your own body or that of your partner's? Hop in the shower together before any below-the-belt action occurs. You can soap up and rub down each others' bodies, make out under the hot water, and write naughty things to each other on the steam in the mirror. Don't forget to clean each other gently between the legs with a good, unscented, pH-balanced soap, and rinse it all away. Bonus: You both know that you're BOTH squeaky clean before sexy and salacious things start to happen, and that means one less thing to be worried about when you go down on each other.

Note: Please don't ever use store-bought douches or scented wipes to try to change the scents of your lovely bits — harsh chemicals and fragrances in these products can seriously mess with both the pH and the natural flora of the vagina, which can result in unwanted infections. If you feel that for some reason you absolutely must douche, please empty out the bottle of its original chemical-filled concoction and refill it with warm water or even warm saltwater. That's more than enough to rinse everything out and keep you from being susceptible to infection in the area that you probably want it least.

Myth

Hair on a vulva/mons pubis/pubic bone is dirty/unhygienic/gross.

Busted

People choose to style their pubic hair in many different ways! Whether someone chooses to let it grow out, trims it evenly, decorates it, dyes it (with pubic hair–friendly dyes — not the usual hair dye!), creates interesting patterns with it, or removes it altogether by shaving, waxing, or sugaring, it's only dirty if someone doesn't take care of themselves by keeping up with their cleanliness. Having pubic hair doesn't mean that someone is dirty, just like shaving doesn't mean someone's clean. Whatever pubic hairstyle (or lack thereof) that you or your partner chooses to rock, embrace it, love it, and get ready to go downtown for some fun action! If you or your partner happens to choose to keep the hair as part of the fun, try using it as part of your oral sex play. Some people enjoy a gentle pull, others like having fingers run through it, and you might even discover something else that you or your partner may enjoy having done to your pubic hair.

On that note, sometimes people worry about their partner ingesting pubic hair while they're getting down and dirty. Never fear — there's a super easy solution that anyone can do at any time, no preparation or props needed. Just run your fingers through your pubic hair (or your partner's) before the action starts, tugging slightly on the hair, as if your fingers were a fancy hairbrush designed just for pubic hair. This'll dislodge and remove any loose hairs so that you can focus on the activity at hand (or at mouth)!

Myth

Oral sex should be done for only a minute or two as foreplay before the "real" stuff begins to happen.

Busted

While cunnilingus can certainly take a starring role in foreplay, it can also be the main event, or even dessert. You can start out with oral, move to something else, and come back to oral, or even spend a fun-filled evening with nothing but an oral sex extravaganza. Oral is its own exciting activity and should never have the word "just" put in front of it, as in "We just had oral sex last night."

Let's give oral the fabulous attention and respect that it deserves as a fun-filled activity by itself, and if other things happen to be on the menu before, during, or even after oral, then so be it.

Another thing to keep in mind is that the arousal in vulva owners (mostly women) is very different than the arousal in penis owners (mostly men). While most people with penises can orgasm from oral sex in anywhere from thirty seconds to ten minutes, those receiving cunnilingus can take twenty to forty minutes (and more!) until the fireworks launch. While there are individual exceptions, plan on spending a good deal of time enjoying your partner's cave of wonders. It's much better to have your partner ask you to stop because you're pleasuring them so much for so long than to have them wonder why oral sex was just a drive-by on the way to other bedroom activities. Show off your skills, and keep 'em coming! (Pun totally intended.)

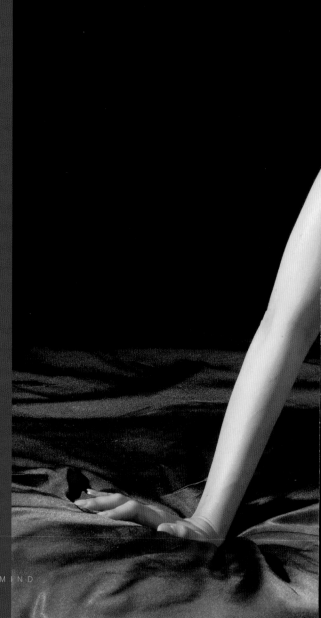

Fulfilling Fantasies

This is a great exercise for partners in a more long-term situation, whether a committed relationship or friends with benefits.

Each of you should sit down and write out your ideal cunnilingus fantasy (yes, the giver can most certainly have a hot cunnilingus fantasy!). If you're not much for writing, perhaps you could record it as an audio file and share it that way. There are no rights or wrongs here; just play out what your ideal going-down situation would be. Is there a particular space that gets you going? Candles? Cars whizzing by? A comfy bed? A bearskin rug? Share every detail you can think of from start to finish. I'm talking about how much time is spent with kissing, what spots of the body are being kissed or are you kissing, how much licking, sucking, fingering, nibbling, and so forth is taking place. What happens in addition to the oral sex, if anything? Get it all out, and then share it with your partner. If you both feel up to it, you can read your fantasies out loud to each other, face-to-face (or play them on the computer/gadget of your choice). If that's a bit too revealing for you, feel free to read it to them over the phone, or even exchange it via e-mail.

While your partner might not be able to go out and get a bearskin rug and fireplace, or spend three days being able to orally worship you, your fantasy will give them a much better idea of some of your turn-ons, what type of

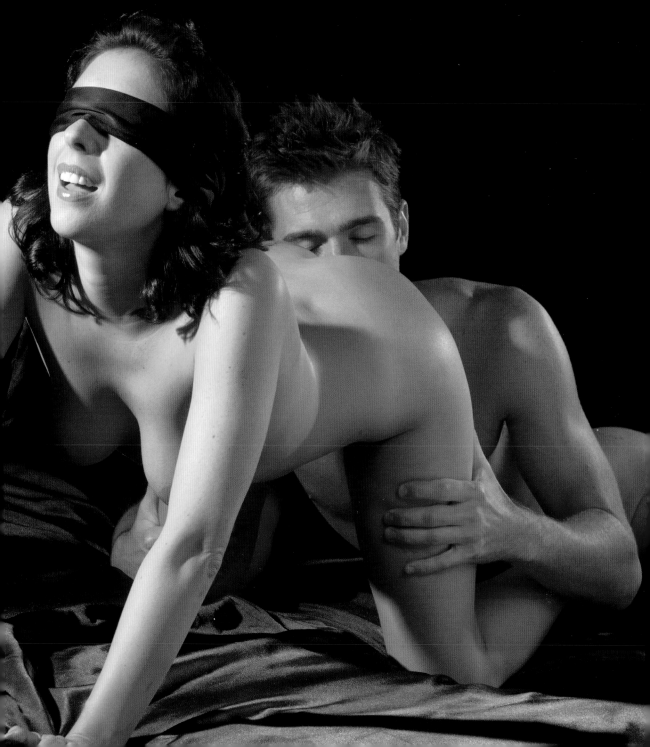

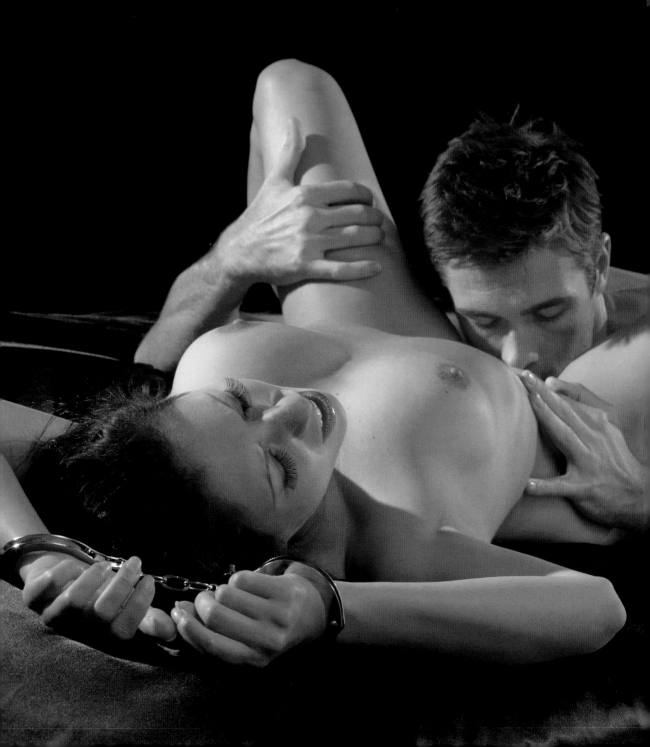

interaction gets you going, and maybe some tidbits to enhance your experience (like a blindfold, certain scented candles, the perfect song on the stereo, etc.). At the very least, it gives each of you a better idea of what feels sexy to YOU; we often don't even spend enough time with ourselves, thinking about what turns us on. If we don't even know our own turn-ons, and our own fantasies, how can we be expected to be able to share them with our partners when asked?

I Want THAT!

Rent or purchase some sexy DVDs, or stream some movies online. They can be soft core or hard core — whatever works best for the two of you. (Note: Plenty of companies make porn where the performers choose their partners and what happens, and these often feel like more authentic experiences of pleasure for the viewers. Some recommendations include Sweetheart Video, Sweet Sinner Video, Femme Production, Comstock Films, Heartcore Productions, Reel Queer Productions, and Pink and White Productions.) Select some scenes that you both find hot and steamy, and share what turns you on about each of them. Is it the eye contact? The positions? The music? Whatever gets you going, share that with your partner, and talk about how you can integrate that into how the two of you get it on.

If visual hotness is not such a good fit for you, check out some erotica books. There's a great variety of anthologies available, some by female authors, some by orientation, and others by fetishes or kinks, or even locations (like the beach) or seasons. Pick out a few, and either read stories out loud to each other or take turns reading them, and leave notes in the margins (or sticky notes on the edges) near things that get your motor going — and then switch. Once you've both read over the raunchy bits, meet up to discuss what you liked best, why you liked it, and how the two of you can add that to your real-life sexy times!

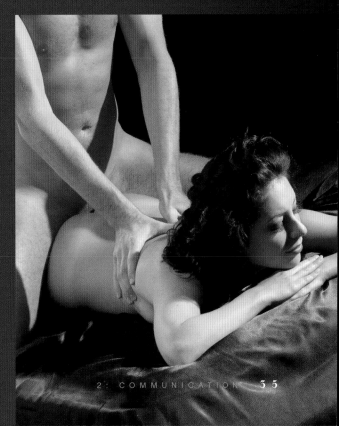

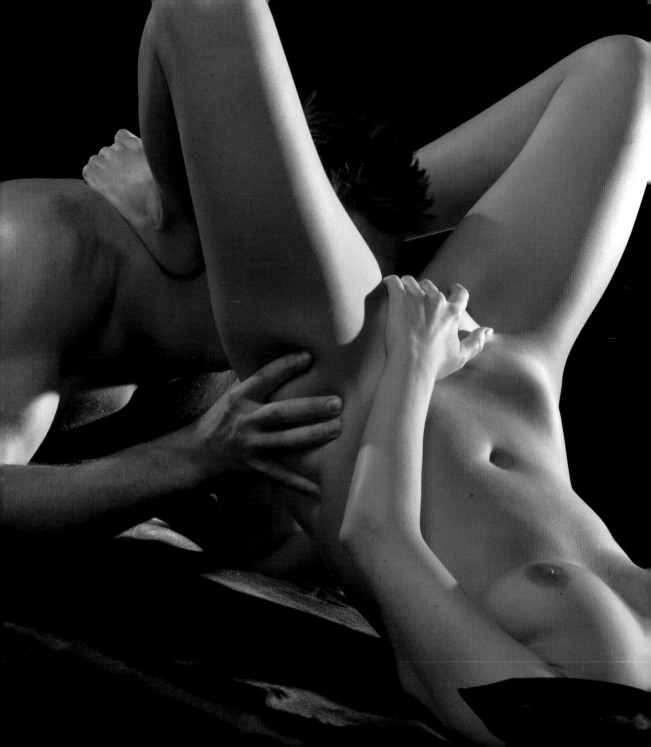

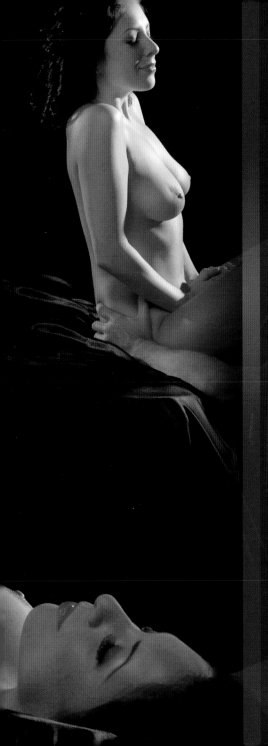

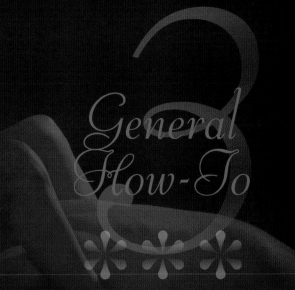

General How-To

We're going to begin at the beginning.
And what better place to start than kissing your partner
. . . ABOVE the waist.

Oftentimes, people get so incredibly excited (and/or
nervous) about going down on their partner that they
rush through the whole process of getting their partner
turned on and getting turned on themselves. While a
few select people can go from zero to OH MY GOD
in sixty seconds, most people like a warm-up before
indulging in the breakfast of champions. Talk to your
partner, and ask them what their idea of a warm-up
is. They might know exactly where they'd like to be
kissed, and that's certainly good information to have.

But maybe no one's ever taken the time to really make them feel good, and your effort to do so will blow their mind.

So sit back, relax a little, and enjoy the entire experience. While you may be ready and raring to go, completely set to dive between their legs and show them how much you appreciate them and their delectable vulva, taking the time to turn them on is what will set you apart. It's far better to tantalize and tease your partner until they're absolutely begging you to go down on them, than to move too quickly and have them pull away because they just aren't ready for that yet. Give them the whole razzle-dazzle, and show them that you care about giving them a great cunnilingus experience. So where to start?

Start High

The head can be an incredibly erogenous place. From kissing their earlobes (and whispering sweet and dirty things in their ears) to kissing and nibbling their sweet lips to gently grazing your lips across their cheek, you can work these sensitive areas until your partner is starting to get fairly hot and heavy. Different people like different things, so experiment and take mental notes on what it is that gets your partner revved up.

How about the neck? Supersexy and full of delicious nerve endings, the neck is a great place to lick, nibble, blow, bite, suck (be careful of bruises/hickies if your partner would prefer

NOT to have them—this is definitely a good conversation to have before things get too hot and heavy), and more. Lots of people like having the front and side of their neck stimulated, while others like having the back of it kissed and loved. You can lick a spot and blow on it for a chilling sensation, or instead of blowing through your whole mouth, you can breathe out on them with warm air, providing a nice warming sensation.

The next stop on the body (although you certainly don't have to do it in any order), is the collar bone, which is incredibly sensitive for most people, as well as the upper arms, which many people like to have rubbed or gently scratched. Spend some time here, kissing, nuzzling, gently nipping—whatever feels good and gets your partner's engine going.

Then there are the breasts! Don't just go in for the kill by moving right to the nipples. We've all heard the joke about lovers twisting the nipples as if they were searching for a radio station. None of that, unless your partner tells you that direct nipple action is what they want. Start out lightly, gently caressing the area all around the nipple, but DO NOT touch the nipple yet. It's much nicer to tease until they can't take it anymore and you just HAVE to touch them than to go too fast, and have them feel like it was a drive-by consensual grope. Some people prefer a firmer touch or grab on their breasts; again, it's absolutely OK to ask what they like and get

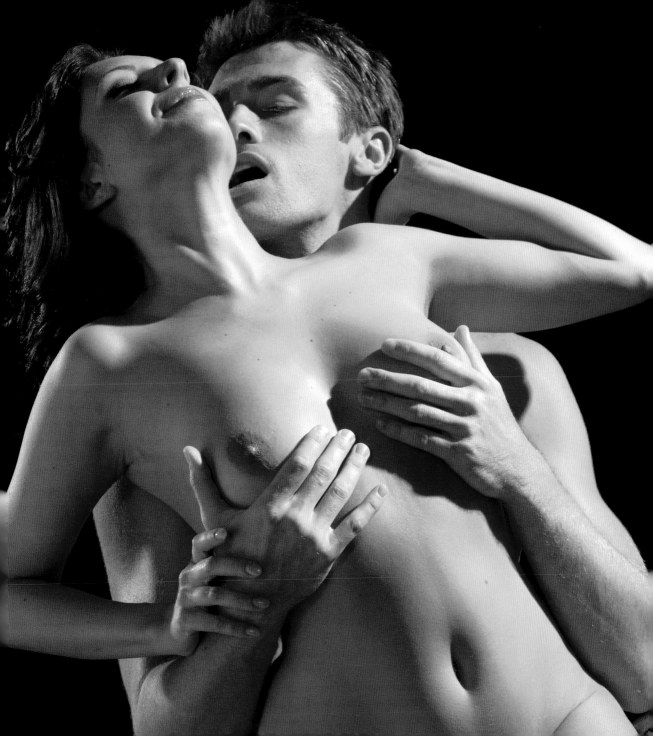

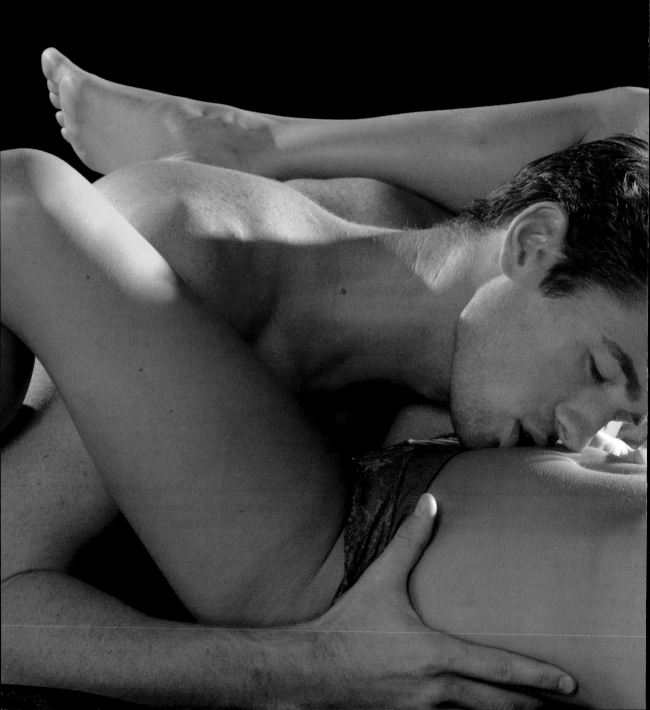

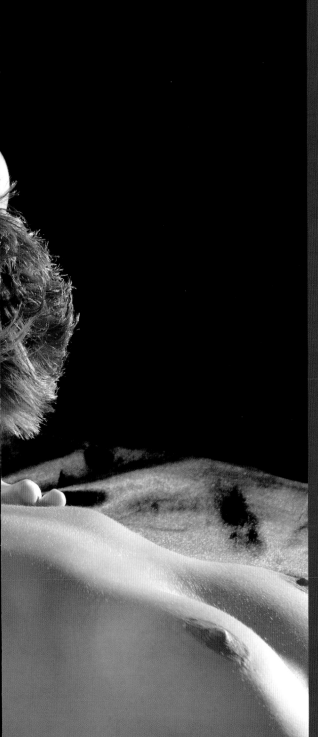

some feedback. Being a good partner sexually is not about being a know-it-all; it's about listening and learning, and continuing to change your game plans based on the feedback received.

Feel around the breasts. Lift them gently, kiss them, nibble on them, and then — finally — time for the nipple loving. You can brush them with your fingers, tease them with your tongue, even give them a teeny nibble with your teeth. Some people like rougher stimulation; if that's the case, then work your way up to the level they like. Others like just a feather touch to tantalize and tease them. Find out what your partner likes and what gets their engine going.

Go Down

A little farther down, the stomach and hip bones are great places to gently stroke and softly kiss as you explore your partner's beautiful skin. For some, the hip bone area is quite ticklish, while for others, that's a direct line to the genitals. Why not find out? It's always possible it's neither for your partner, so don't put all your eggs in one basket; keep exploring their body to figure out their different erogenous zones, and keep mixing it up.

Let's skip the vulva for now, and enjoy those long and luscious legs. Lots and lots of people love having their thighs, especially their inner thighs, kissed, licked, rubbed, bitten, and more. Explore and enjoy the experience as you get your partner close to the edge of pleasure. If our partner likes more sensation play, consider running your nails down their inner thighs, or bringing in a feather tickler to add some different sensations.

Having taken the time to warm up your partner and explore their pleasure zones, you can now start honing in on the main event (at least as far as this book is concerned): cunnilingus! Placing gentle kisses on the mons (pubic bone) as well as rubbing it with the palm of your hand can build up even more anticipation as well as feel incredibly delightful to your partner. Again, watch them for body language and listen for feedback. It'll help you learn which stimulations and sensations they like and which they couldn't care less about.

Gently (or aggressively, if that's how you both want to play), open your partner's legs. Stop for a moment. Yes, you want to dive in. Yes, you want to give your partner as much pleasure as they can possibly handle. But wait a moment. Take a look at their vulva, how beautiful and unique it is, and let them know that you find it hot and sexy. Lots of people have never even seen their own vulvas, and there's a lot of shame over female genitalia. But if you can show your partner how amazing you find them, and how much you want to enjoy your time below the belt, it can help them feel infinitely more comfortable. Check out the section on vulvar viewing for some tips on how to go all out on vulva appreciation time.

Dive In

So you've taken your vulva-gazing break. Fabulous. Now the time has come to go in for some stimulating action. Again, start slow. Most (although not all) people don't like to have their clit be the first thing stimulated. It can be incredibly sensitive, and starting there won't always feel good or may feel a little too intense. Luckily, you can start by playing with the inner and outer labia, gently stimulating the clitoral hood with your fingers and more. Think of the clit as the center of a spiral or bull's-eye, and imagine that you have to work your way through all the outside layers before you can go to town on the central area. Your hands can be magical things, as long as you take the time to learn how to use them properly.

In movies, we tend to see folks just shoving their hands down their partner's panties, hunting around as if searching for the power button that they can push to make the geyser of pleasure start. While this may seem to make sense to some people, many folks with vulvas don't appreciate how this feels. Many prefer the vulva to be treated sensually and with gentler action, so after you kiss your way up your partner's thighs and are in the middle of the special zone, take your time, take a deep breath, and remember that the weight of the world is not resting on your shoulders. Success doesn't ride on whether you can stimulate the clitoris in the quickest way possible; it rides on

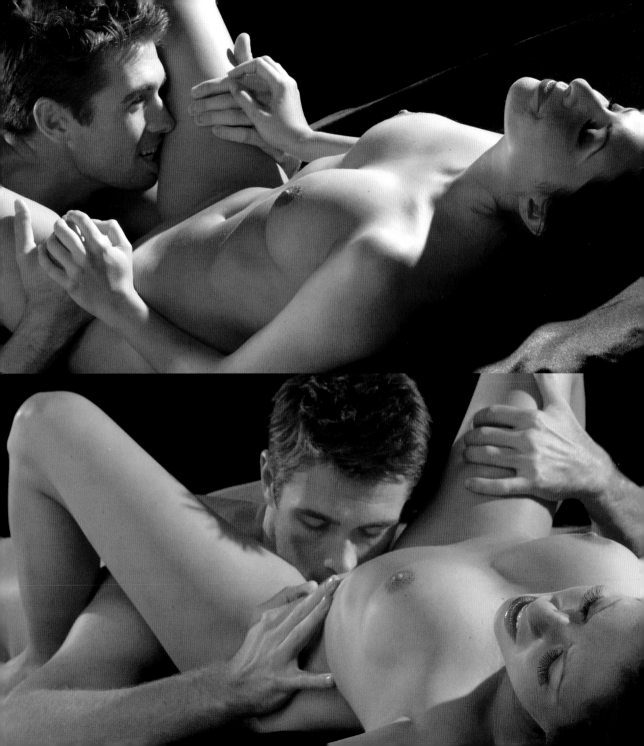

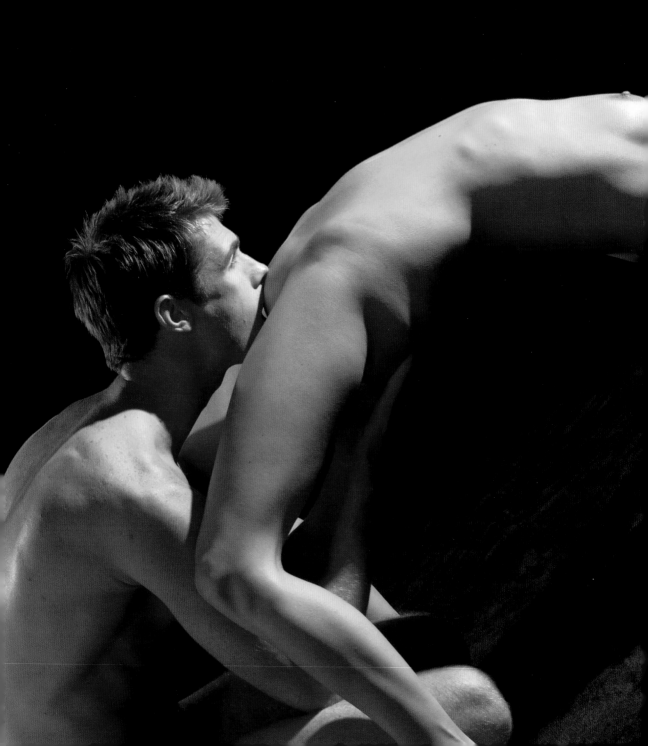

whether you and your partner are both having fun throughout the experience.

If your partner's genitals are not yet lubricated or don't have enough lubrication to keep things fun, slippery, and sliding, then this is an ideal time to add lube. Check out the lubrication section for more information on the perfect match of lubricant for you. This might also be a good time to have your partner show you how they enjoy being touched. Try having your hand over theirs, or vice versa, as they move it around and show you their favorite pleasurable areas. If you're up for it, this is also a great time to watch them masturbate with a sex toy, perhaps using a simple vibrator to warm the area up while you watch them and enjoy the sexy show unfolding in front of you. Maybe you could even take control of the vibrator and use it to provide a little extra boost of pleasure before you go in for some delicious licking.

Slowly and gently rub your entire hand up and down the vulva, making sure to touch both sets of the labia (lips) and the clitoris. Remember, it's much more fun to start slowly and have your partner begging you to ramp up your ministrations than it is to have them ask you to slow down or stop because things got too intense too quickly. Once you've given the entire vulva area a lot of love with your whole hand, spread your fingers as you continue to stroke your hand up and down, letting them naturally fall into the folds of the vulva, providing additional

stimulation to your partner. If they're ready fo it, you can use a lubricated fingertip to stimulate the clitoral hood from the outside — remember do NOT actually go straight for the clit. It needs to be wooed and can take a bit more time to ge ready for the action at hand (or at mouth, as the case may be). You can provide this handiwork in any sort of position, from spooning in bed to lying between your partner's legs, even to standing up and being face-to-face or reaching around. Mix things up, and do whatever feels good (or fun!) for the two of you. After you fee as if you've given the vulva enough time with your fabulous fingers, it's time to turn to you tongue and let your partner feel your desire through the amazing action you're about to give them. Let's get to the licking!

Licking

Take your time. It's different for each person and could be anywhere from a minute or two to half an hour (or more) before your partner is ready for action on the clit. While everybody's unique, many studies have shown that most women would like more time spent on them during cunnilingus, between fifteen and forty-five minutes more than what they're already getting. Of course, maybe this doesn't apply to YOUR situation (there are always some folks who want less teasing, warm-up, and foreplay and just want you to dive right in), but it's a good guide for people wondering how long they should take on going down. There isn't a magic number, but most people want more than they're getting. Communicate with your partner to get their feelings on this, but as a general rule, if you think you've licked enough, keep on licking, and then . . . lick some more!

When it comes to licking, you can do all kinds of things with your tongue. Stick it out of your mouth right now—doesn't matter where you are. Flatten it out and make it as wide as you can. A lick like this is à la Shirley Temple licking a giant lollipop. Now make it pointy. A lick with your tongue like this is much more direct and intense.

Do some tongue exercises; move it side to side, in and out, up and down, in a circle, back and forth. Keep doing that until it gets tired. This is a great set of exercises for when you're studying for a final, are bored at your desk in your office, or are stuck in traffic. Your tongue is a muscle, too; the more you work it out, the more you build up that muscle (plain ol' talking does count) and the less likely it'll tire out during cunnilingus. Sound silly? Perhaps. But great athletes exercise even while not actively playing, and even crossword puzzle champions practice with the *New York Times* Sunday crossword. Taking a bit of extra time out of your week to work on strengthening your tongue, and experimenting with different ways of using it, can definitely elevate you in the world of cunnilingus givers. It shows that you're willing to take some time and work to bring yourself to a different level.

Different people like different licks, and they like them at different times of cunnilingus. Usually,

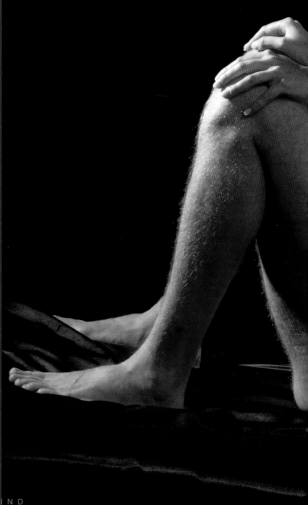

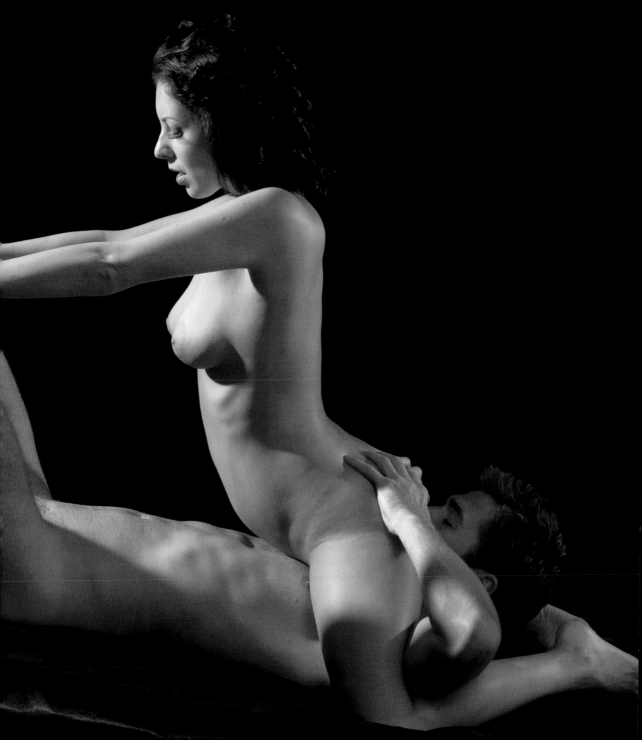

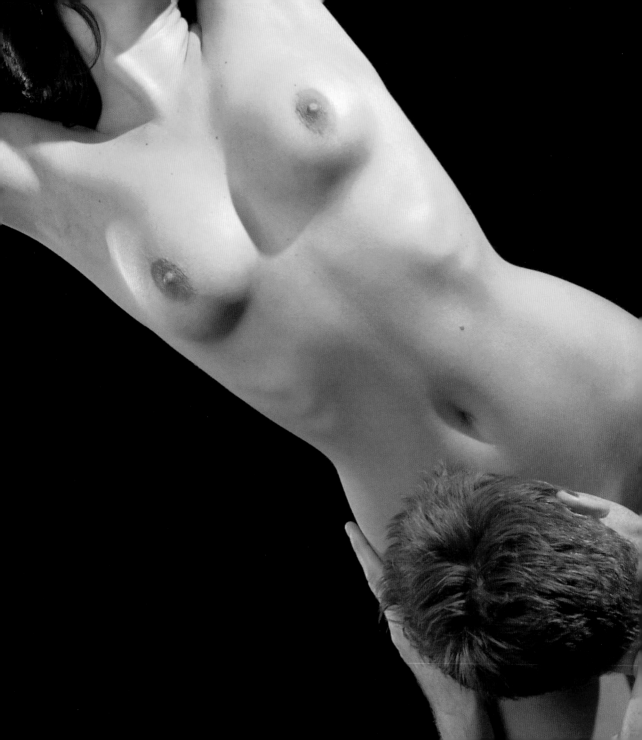

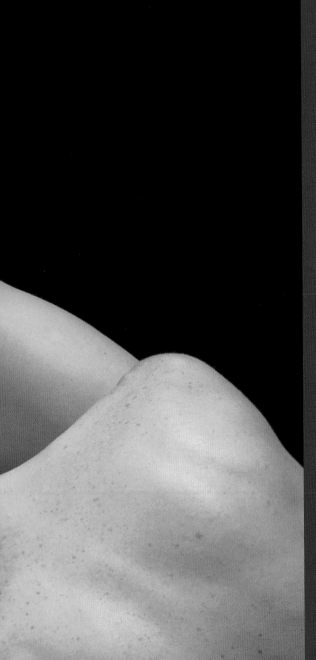

starting with a flat tongue to get a more diffuse sensation is perfect in the beginning, while a more pointed and direct tongue can provide the stimulation to bring it home toward the end. Feel free to mix up the licks, too, especially early on, when you're trying out different kinds of sensations to warm up your partner and see what they like. As your partner gets closer to orgasm (if that's your shared goal), stick with the lick they like.

Frequently, cunnilingus givers think that their partner might be getting bored with the licking, and change up their licking pattern right before orgasm. For some people, this can be incredibly frustrating. A good way to handle this is to have a sign, like having the receiver tap the bed, or pull the giver's hair, or squeeze the giver's shoulders when an orgasm is getting close. This way, the giver knows to bring it home with the same type of licking sensation, instead of choosing that moment to change it up.

Not sure what kind of lick your partner likes? Try a bunch and ask them to tell you, to moan loudly, or to tap your head or shoulder when you do something that feels good. If you want to make it a little silly, or bring in some hot and fun medical role play, you can do the "optometrist" move. You know: "Which do you like better? Number 1 or number 2? Number 2 or number 3?" and so on. A little ridiculous? Yes, but it can be a ton of fun, and you'll be able to figure out what your partner likes easily. If you like,
(text continued on p. 52)

Lubrication

One of the great rules of amazing sex is that Lube Is Love. In case you missed it, let's say it together: Lube Is Love!

Why should lube matter? Lubrication makes all touch feel better, both outside on the lips, clitoris, and hood and inside the vagina, whether you're using fingers, tongues, or toys. It helps reduce friction, and any testing of your own will probably demonstrate that vulvas prefer slippery, slidey sensations to those that produce friction and drag. Lube can help transmit sensations better and can also reduce the amount of work to be done by the person performing oral sex and manual stimulation. Also, if you're using fingers or toys in the vagina, using lube will help prevent or reduce soreness as well as prevent tearing of the delicate vaginal tissue. Any way you look at it, lube is pretty amazing.

Most vulvas lubricate naturally to some extent, with some tending to provide more natural lubrication than others. The amount of lube produced by a vulva doesn't always have a direct correlation to how turned on the person is; a person can be raring to go but have little to no lubricant being produced, while someone else has a river of natural lubrication, and all they're thinking about is what they forgot to set up on their DVR. Don't use lubrication as an indication of arousal. Just ask your partner how they're feeling, if they're turned on, and if they're ready for you to do deliciously dirty things to them. Going by those answers tends to be a much better estimation of their arousal level.

While vulvas tend to lubricate on their own, many things can affect natural lubrication, effectively drying up the vulva. These external influences can include hormonal birth control (the patch, the pill, the ring, the Implanon, the shot, etc.), antihistamines (any allergy medication, both prescription and over the counter), and stress (which tends to affect anyone who's capable of breathing). Because all of these things can dry up lubrication, and the fact that sometimes a sex session can last for hours on end, beyond the vulva's traditional lubrication cycle, it's always good to have some vulva-friendly lube on hand. Pun intended.

What makes a lubricant vulva friendly? Well, first of all, it should not have ANY oil or petroleum product in the ingredient list. Think about your hands when you're washing dishes; if you get a layer of oil on them, water just beads up on your hands until you use a hard-core grease-cutting soap to clean up. Same goes for the vagina. If you put an oil-based lube (or lotion, or cooking oil, etc.) in the vaginal canal, it'll coat the walls of the vagina. This is bad, because the vagina cleans itself through transudation, where fluid comes through the vaginal walls, like an overfilled sponge. If you coat the walls with oil or oil-like substances, you prevent the vagina from cleaning itself. This means it's now more susceptible to infections, and that's not fun. Keep oil away from the cooch, and everyone's going to be happier.

This leaves two types of lubrications that are friendly for the vagina. The first is silicone-based lubricant. Some well-known brands include Wet Platinum, Eros Bodyglide, Pjur, Bodyglide, Gun Oil (not actually oil based), and Pink. Silicone lube is friendly for the vagina, but isn't compatible with silicone toys, or any soft, squishy toy. It also, while not poisonous, is not the tastiest of lubes. This might be a great lube to use for manual stimulation prior to, during, or after oral sex (or on its own!), vaginal intercourse, anal stimulation, anal intercourse, hand jobs, and so forth. It's also completely compatible with any type of condoms, gloves, and dams.

The second type of lubricant is also the most well-known; it's water-based lubricant. Some well-known vulva-friendly brands include Sliquid, Maximus, Wet Naturals, Pink Water, and Blossom Organics. Water-based lube is compatible with all types of toys, with all types of condoms, gloves, and dams, and with most bodies. But some of the flavored water-based lubricants contain sugar. NEVER use a lubricant with sugar in it near the vulva: that's basically asking for a yeast infection. Sugary lubes are usually sold for novelty use only, and while great for blow jobs, they should be kept away from the vagina and the anus. Another ingredient in many water-based lubes is glycerin. Glycerin is a safe ingredient overall — it's used in many health and beauty products. But many vulvas seem to have a negative reaction to glycerin; in some folks, it can cause itching or allergic reactions, while others can experience yeast infections or irritation. If you or your partner ever has these sensations after using a water-based lubricant that contains glycerin, try out a glycerin-free option.

How much lube should you use? As much as you want! Keeping the vulva wet and slippery is the name of the game, so add as much as you'd like. With silicone-based lube, it keeps going and going and going, so you probably won't need to reapply or reactivate. With water-based lube, it can dry up as it gets used. For most people, their first inclination is to add more. The problem with that is the lube may get stickier and stickier. You can actually reactivate water-based lube by adding more water. You can do this by spitting, by pouring a little water from a cup, glass, or bottle, by hopping in the shower, or by using a mister or squirt gun.

Some people think that if flavored lube is a good idea (which it definitely can be), other things can double for this, like chocolate syrup, whipped cream, sweet liqueurs, and so forth. The problem is that all of these things contain sugar. To repeat: placing sugar on, near, in, or anywhere about the vulva is basically an open invitation for a yeast infection. I'm not saying that you absolutely CANNOT eat an ice cream sundae off of your partner's vulva, but if you want to do so, I'd suggest using a layer of plastic kitchen wrap between the vulva and the sugary concoction. Either that, or be prepared for a gynecologist's visit and a round of antibiotics.

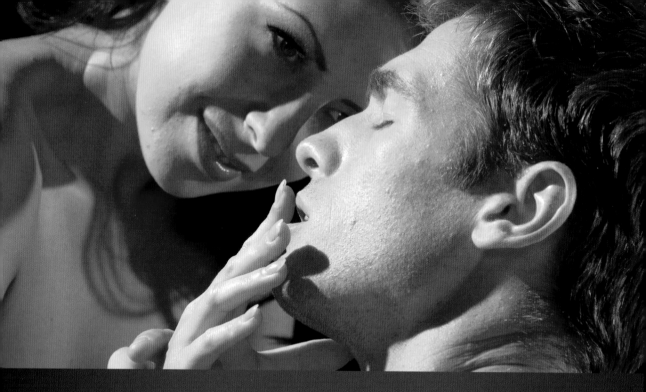

you can name different licks that your partner enjoys. That way, if they'd like to request the tongue tornado followed by the floppy flip, you'll both know what they're talking about, and you have some good direction to go with your licking patterns.

A–Z

Almost everyone who talks about learning to lick brings up the alphabet trick, telling you to lick in the shape of A to Z with your tongue. Now, this both has merit and is kind of ridiculous. If you just lick through the alphabet without pause, you're going to be providing all sorts of different sensations to your partner one right after another with no break in between — and they're going to love some and hate others. How much does that suck when your partner gives you exactly the right sensation to get you going . . . and then switches to another? Frustrating, right? Even more so when you're not sure which sensation was which letter, so you can't ask for the one that felt best. Never fear; here are some ideas that might help!

A better way to do this is to experiment one letter at a time, or maybe try out a few words, and ask for their input. Don't forget that each letter has FOUR shapes: uppercase scripts, lowercase script, uppercase block, and lowercase block.

This means you have ninety-six different letter options, and don't even get me started on numbers, symbols, and more. Take it easy on the A to Z and just start with ABC or XYZ until you figure out which letters get your partner's hips bucking. As you spend more time down under with them, you can try out different letters or add the cursive alphabet, until you can write them love letters on their vulva with the tip of your tongue. Now, that's definitely an exaggeration (until someone tries it and tells me how awesome it is), but it's a good idea to start slowly with only a few variations done slowly (to allow your partner to give accurate feedback) and to work your way up from there.

Geometric Shapes

In the same vein as the ABCs, you can also make different geometric shapes on and around the vulva before you. Whether your choice is a box around the box, or concentric circles growing closer and closer, different shapes provide you with the option to get feedback from your partner, and the ability to add their favorite shape or shapes to your repertoire. You can choose to make larger shapes like circles or squares that encompass the vulva's entire outer rim, or smaller ones that go across the middle for a moment or two. If you're into fun games during sexy time, why not ask your partner to guess which shape it is that's making them squirm? Just be nice, and don't hit them with

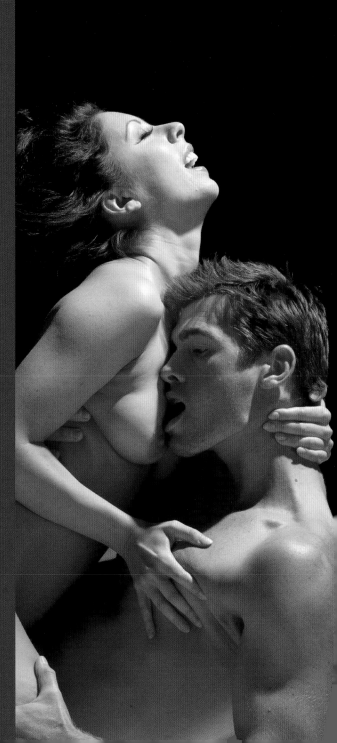

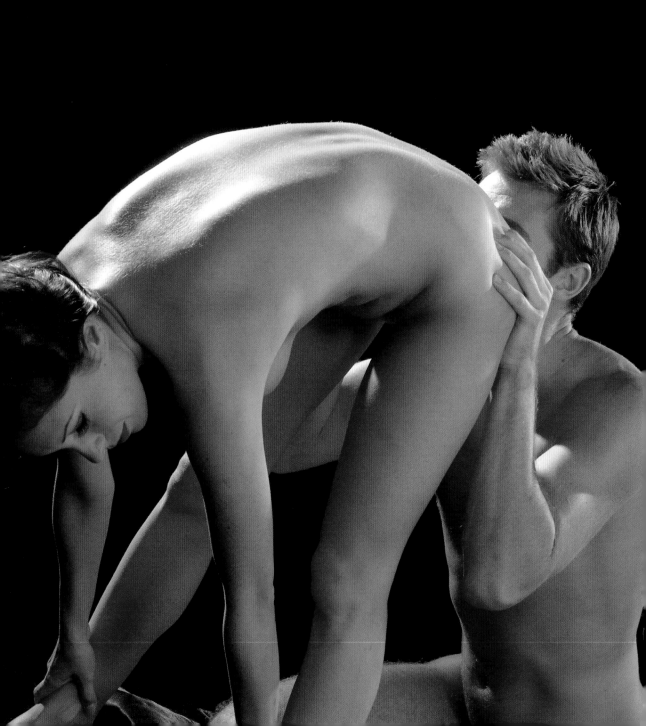

a tetrahedron . . . unless of course you're role-playing Math Professor and Naughty Student.

Doggy Licks

Have you ever seen a big ole slobbery dog with its tongue hanging out of its mouth, covered with saliva, ready to lick the first human, bone, or Popsicle it comes across? As silly as it might sound, channel that hound! Especially early on in cunnilingus, using a big, slobbery, flat tongue to lick all around the vulva area can serve multiple purposes. First, it can help you get the entire area nice and moist, which makes everything else you're about to do feel that much better. Second, a big, flat tongue full of saliva will allow you to cover more area, allowing you to stimulate all of the different nerve endings around the vulva. Lastly, with the lubrication from your saliva and the flatness of your tongue, this stimulation is gentler, which is ideal for the type of stimulation most receivers enjoy earlier on in their cunnilingus experience.

A problem that many people have while giving oral sex (either cunnilingus or fellatio) is their concern about looking good. This concern frequently has them sucking in all of their spit and saliva and swallowing it, rather than putting it to good use. Now, I'm not suggesting that you spit on your partner in the middle of oral sex (unless that's something that you've both discussed previously, or they ask you to do so while in the throes of passion), but in cunnilingus, wetter is better! Let that spit and saliva drip right out of your mouth and onto the glorious vulva in front of you. Wetness, whether from natural lubrication, saliva, or added lubrication, is crucial to any stimulation of the vulva. That wetness reduces drag from your tongue, fingers, and anything else that you might be using to stimulate the vulva. Less friction equals a lot more fun, and more good feelings on the receiver's part. So stop sucking up your saliva and awkwardly trying to swallow in the middle of hot oral sex; just let it go, and put it to good use!

Anywhere but There

Don't forget to take your time. Whether you choose to lick around the vulva in a clocklike motion or provide random licking and sucking, make sure to explore all the different erotic sensations provided by the areas that are not the clitoris, or even the clitoral hood. The more you explore around the vulva, and lick, touch, and suck, the more aroused your partner will get. By the time you're finally making your way to the middle, and getting ready to give your ministrations to the clit, your partner might be begging you to do so. Feel free to make them beg a bit more or to choose to satisfy them right away. Either way, you've helped raise their level of pleasure, making whatever will end your playtime (an orgasm from cunnilingus, or moving on to something else) that much more intense as the endorphins are cruising through their system. And the more time you spend timulating them anywhere but the clitoris, the more you learn about their body and the pleasure they like.

Givers of cunnilingus tend to go straight for the clit. Now, please don't get me wrong, the clit is amazing. But it's not the magic go button that society often says that it is. If there isn't adequate warm up of the person and their body, focusing too much attention on the clit too soon can feel way too intense for some folks and can even be painful to others. Take your time, and if you don't have much experience with your partner, let them guide you as to when it's time to give the clit your undivided attention. Is clitoral stimulation a big part of cunnilingus for most folks? Absolutely. Just make it a fun-filled journey to get there, instead of seeing it as the main goal, and I guarantee, both of you will have a much better time than if you just lock your sights on it and blow past everything else to get there.

Fire and Ice

Many people love to play with temperatures, and this can be a great way to mix things up during cunnilingus. If your partner is sensitive to temperature, or happens to not like surprises, it would be smart to let them know in advance that you plan to start playing around with different temperatures.

Making your mouth cold is quite simple: take a cold drink of water, or suck on an ice cube,

and voila! A self-cooled mouth in no time. I will caution you that while it might sound like a supersexy idea to suck on a delicious Popsicle and then go down on your partner, this probably isn't the most brilliant thing to do. Most Popsicles contain sugars, and that means that you'd be transferring sugars to your partner's vulva, which usually results in a yeast infection. Stick with sugar-free Popsicles, or the oh-so-easy-to-find ice cubes, and you'll be able to cool down your mouth in a jiffy in a way that's friendly to your partner's vulvar flora. You can even use a melty ice cube to stimulate them directly; just make sure it's melted a bit before using it, so that you don't accidently end up with tongue-on-frozen-pole syndrome with the delicate vulva.

As far as heating things up, taking a sip of warm water or tea can help warm up your mouth without getting it too hot. Taking a gulp of peppermint herbal tea can even mix warming sensations with tingling sensations, all without involving sugar. Other people have suggested breath mints, crème de menthe liqueur, and dissolving breath strips; I'd definitely check on the sugar content first before trying these out. At least if you make the herbal tea, you know there's no chance of accidentally putting sugar near the vulva. Also, some people have sensitivities to mint; ask your partner before you add a hint of mint to your sex life. An accidental sex-driven trip to the doctor is no fun and it totally kills the mood.

If you're heating up or cooling down sex toys, always do so in a bowl of warm water or ice water. Never put a toy in the freezer before using it on a person, and never boil or microwave a toy before using it on a person. A little bit goes a long way in temperature play with the naughty bits; it's always easier to go cooler or warmer next time than to deal with a frostbitten or singed vulva.

Freestyle Licking

Sometimes, we read too much, watch too many educational sex DVDs, and allow advice from our friends and ex-partners to overstimulate our brains while we're trying to stimulate the delicious and exciting vulva at hand. You can lick until you're blue in the face (no, this doesn't actually happen) or until your tongue falls out (no, this one doesn't happen either, I promise), but if you're spending the whole time running through tips and tidbits, you might be shooting yourself in the foot. Being present in your sexual activity is an incredibly important part of being enthusiastic, and as I've discussed already, enthusiasm is a huge part of providing enjoyable cunnilingus, for both parties involved.

So yes, read your books, and go through this one a few times to get yourself comfortable with all of the tricks, tips, techniques, and information. Check out your favorite sex ed scene on the DVD player, and read the erotica that gets your engine going. But once you've gotten to the point where you have pussy in front of your

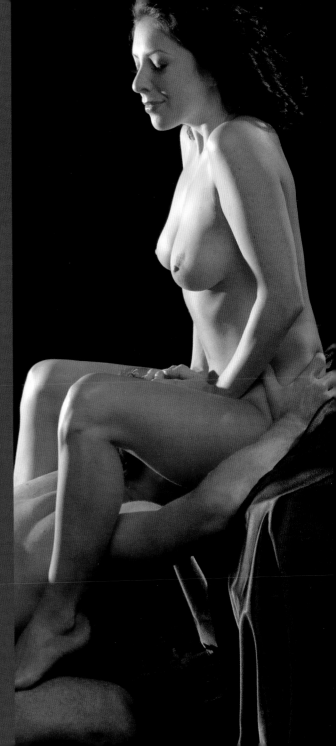

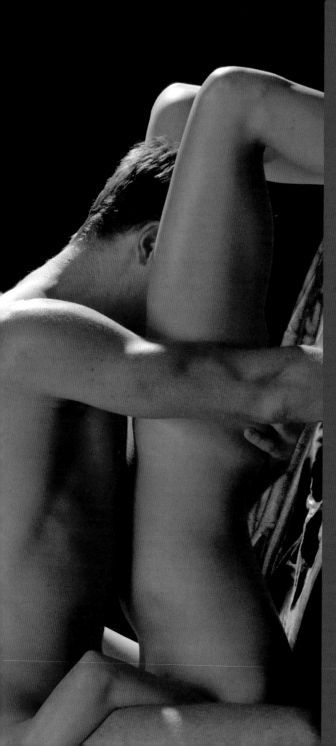

face, enjoy that moment, relax, and do what feels right. If you spend the whole time spelling out your favorite words, or jumping up to make mint tea and grabbing bowls of ice cubes, it's going to mess with the mood, same as if you were counting the licks out loud to make sure you were doing a certain number of each kind. Try out one or two new things per sex session, and also make sure you stick with the moves that are tried and true and that help you stay relaxed, comfortable, and ready for fun.

When you have fun, it's far more likely that your partner is going to have fun, and that's what makes for enjoyable sex of any kind. If your mind goes blank while you're licking that kitty, that's A-OK. This is where "freestyle" licking comes in; just go for it. Do your favorite licks, try anything that occurs to you, or ask your partner what they'd like to experience. Whatever it is, it's sure to be pleasurable on some level, and you can use your partner's feedback to calibrate if you need to be harder or softer, faster or slower, in one spot or in a different one. The only thing that'll stress you out is if you freeze up. But knowing that you can always turn to the exciting world of freestyle licking means that you don't have to be concerned with a brain fart midlick. If it happens, go freestyle, and really strut your stuff.

Let's Get a Little More Hands-on

While you're using your oh-so-talented tongue to provide amazing oral action all around and up and down the vulva, it's more than just OK to also use your hands as tools of pleasure. You may be in a position that requires you to use your hands to support yourself or your partner, or maybe you're using them to help hold legs open or to keep your head comfortable. If so, that's fine, feel free to skip ahead. But it's likely that at some point during cunnilingus, you'll have an extra free hand or even two. Let's put them to good use!

Remember all of those fun and sexy places we touched on the way to the vulva before diving in? Guess what—you can continue to provide various types of stimulation to these erogenous zones while you're going to town down below! Depending on your current position, you could reach up and play with your partner's breasts and nipples. You could run your fingers (and possibly nails) up and down their thighs and legs, and over their hip bones. Maybe, if they like it, you could reach up and pull their hair, or even just run your fingers through it. Some people like to touch their partner in many ways while giving oral; perhaps reaching up or down and grabbing your partner's hand while going down on them could make the experience even better for them. If you're not sure what might feel good to your partner, just ask! They might have some new and different ideas that will get their engine revving while you work underneath the hood.

Some people may enjoy a bit of penetration vaginally or anally while they're receiving cunnilingus. It's absolutely OK to ask about this and see what they might like. You can use your fingers, or toys, or a combo, to provide this type of stimulation. For more info on toys, check out the sex toy section. If you're putting your fingers in someone, make sure you don't have any sharp nails, rough edges, hang nails, and so forth (and if you do, just use a glove! Check out the section on safer sex). Feel free to add some lube to get things nice and slippery. Start slowly with one or two fingers, and work your way up only if your partner wants more. Some people like in and out stimulation, while others just like having something inside them to squeeze down on, and still others like to have their G-spot stimulated in that "come here" motion. Your partner might not even know what they want; that's fine, because it means you can have fun figuring it out together!

It's possible that your partner might want anal stimulation (either with your fingers or with a toy) while they're receiving head. If so, check out some of the anal toys in the sex toy section, or if you're using your fingers, make sure to wear a glove, or wash your hands thoroughly with soap and warm water before touching the vulva again (the vulva and anus have different bacteria, and anal bacteria can cause vulvar infections if transferred). ALWAYS use lube with any type of anal stimulation or penetration, because the anus doesn't produce any lube of its own.

You can also use your hands around, in addition to, or in lieu of your tongue when taking a much-needed break. Use lube to make sure things still feel as slippery and slidey as with your tongue, and use your finger(s) to gently play with all of the vulva's fabulous parts: the inner and outer labia, the entrance to the vaginal canal, the mons pubis, the clitoral hood, and yes, even the clitoris. Giving your tongue a break while continuing to provide satisfying stimulation to the vulva can give you a chance to stretch a little, and get into your second, third, or even fourth wind!

This may also be a time to talk about adding some sex toys to the action to add a bit of spice, make things easier for you, and provide multiple types of sensations. There's a whole section on sex toys coming up, but some ideas could include having your lover wear a butt plug during cunnilingus, you wearing a vibrator, cock ring, or butt plug, either or both of you wearing nipple clamps, and any other combo of the above! Adding sex toys doesn't mean anything negative about your superb sexy skill set; it just means that you're open-minded enough to try out all the various things that can add new dimensions to your already rocking sex life!

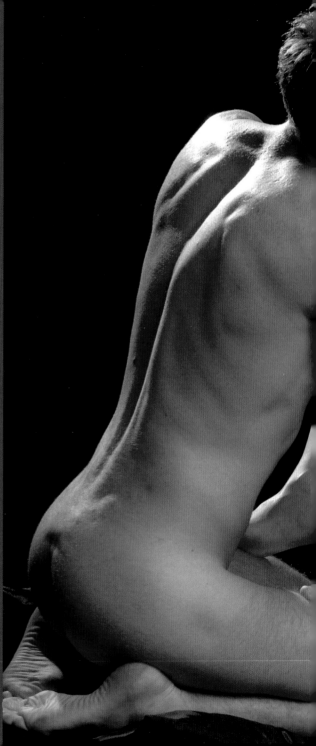

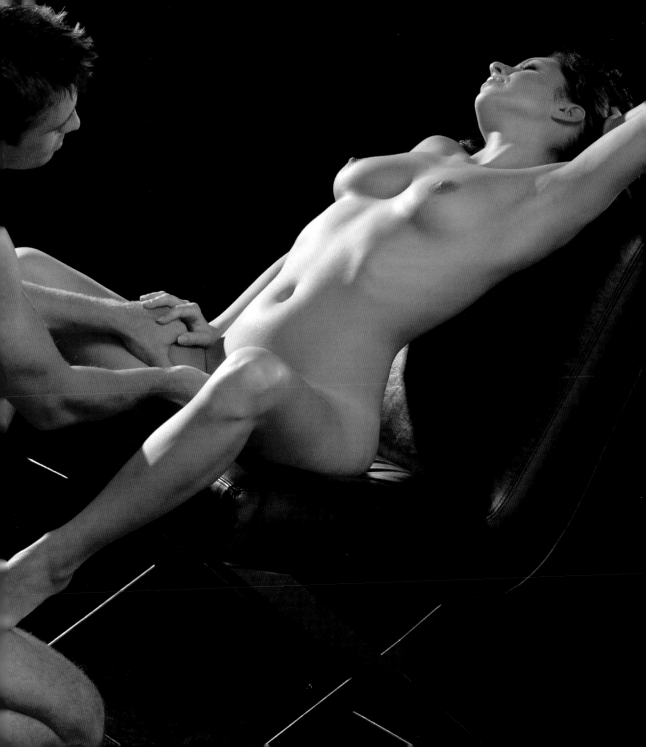

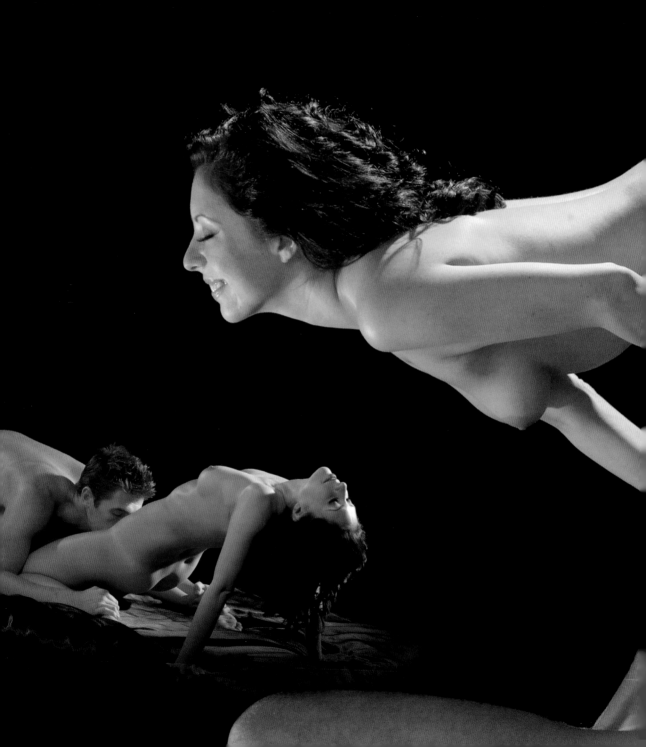

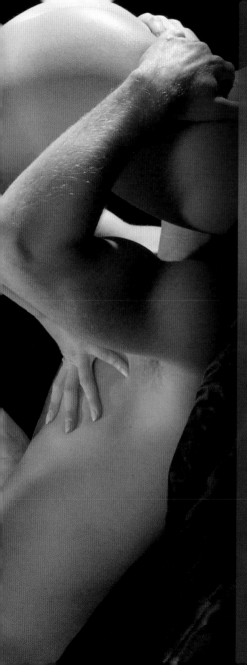

4

Positions

❋ ❋ ❋

*One exciting aspect of cunnilingus
that definitely doesn't get as much
attention as it deserves is the choosing
and using of positions.* There are dozens
of fabulous, comfy, advanced, traditional, and new
positions available for use before, during, and after this
fun-filled act of oral sex. While most people have one
specific position in mind (woman on her back with her
legs spread, possibly knees bent up, her partner on their
stomach, neck craned, between her legs), there are
countless more positions that can be practiced during
your sexy time, that will add pleasure and enjoyment to
the act of cunnilingus.

eed to have a certain number of positions used in every single sex session, that they have to be exactly like the book tells them (or just like in the supersexy movie they have just watched or re still watching), and that they need to be in shape, superflexible, and so on and so on. I'm here to tell you that all of that is simply not true!

The fun of having options means that you can mix things up and keep the spark going, even if you're a longtime cunnilingus devotee. It means that if your neck is getting tired or you're getting a cramp in your leg, you can switch it up, and

your partner have been practicing yoga for the past few months, new positions can give you a sexual challenge, as well as a way to show off all of that hard-earned flexibility. Whatever reason YOU have to try out some new positions is more than good enough for me . . . and if you and your partner are 100 percent satisfied with your current menu of positions, feel free to skip this section. Who am I to mess with a good thing?

First, we'll take a look at some of the more basic, tried-and-true positions for cunnilingus. Some of these you have maybe seen or done before; check them out and make them a little fresher

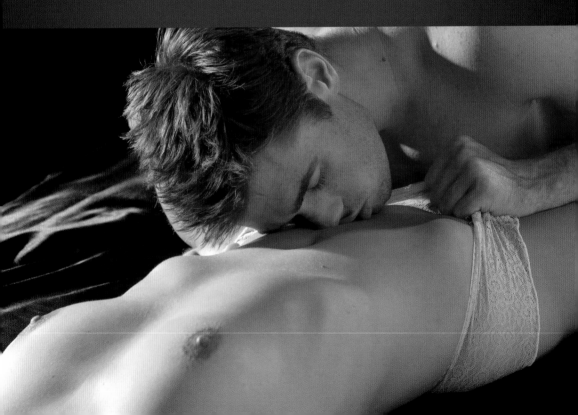

by changing leg, arm, or head positioning, or adding some pillows or furniture. Mixing things up is a good way to start things off and a great way to put a new spin on positions you're already comfortable with.

Once you've gone though the first few positions, the levels will increase slowly. Each position has a level, to give you an idea of how difficult the position might be. Again, there's absolutely no shame in loving positions with lower levels, yet there's nothing to stop you from trying out some of the higher-level positions and laughing alongside your partner if things don't go as planned. Just make sure that if you or your lover has joint, hip, knee, or back problems, that you both aim for positions that aren't going to put any additional stress on these areas. Having to ice various body parts during post-coital cuddle time is not most people's idea of the perfect ending to fabulous sexy time.

The final positions are often referred to as "68" or "69" positions, where both partners get to enjoy oral sex at the same time. But these positions can be a little trickier, for a few reasons. First, it's incredibly difficult for two people to orgasm at the same time, so this can be frustrating if that's your goal. Additionally, it's important to make sure that both of you are careful about the location of your teeth while participating in any 68 or 69 position, because when one partner orgasms, they may clench down with their teeth

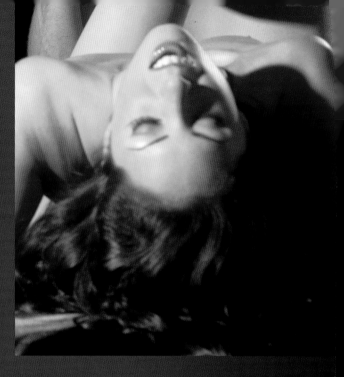

and jaw, which likely will not feel so good to the other partner.

There are many other things you can do to incorporate kink play, power play, sex toys, and more. Trying out the different 68 and 69 positions are great examples of how you can add this type of fun while still keeping things easy and playful. Don't forget that it's always OK to talk about something or suggest it; whether you and your partner decide to try it out is up to the two of you!

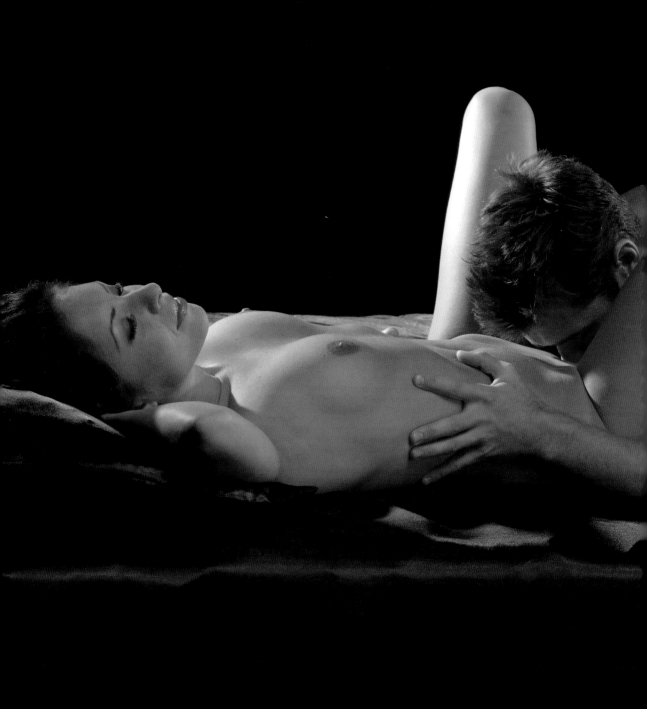

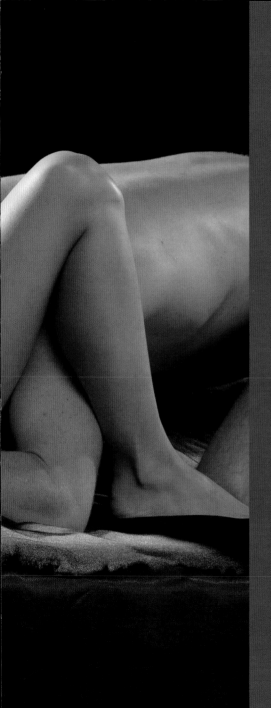

Easy as Pie

In this classic position—the one most people think of when they think of going down—the woman is on her back with her legs spread. Her legs can be either flat on the bed or bent at the knees with her feet flat on the bed/floor/couch. Her partner lies between her legs, face buried in her pussy and arms around her legs.

Level: Any, but great for beginners

Degree of difficulty: 1

Pros: Many women find this to be the best position (or at least one of the best) to climax in. It's pretty easy to get in and out of this position, and it creates little strain on any body parts for either partner. The addition of pillows can change up all the angles, and the woman can control access by closing/opening her legs, and bending/straightening her legs.

Cons: As the classic cunnilingus position, it can feel tired or overused. The partner's neck can often cramp from spending too much time in this position.

Classy Chassis

The woman is on the bed/floor/couch on her hands and knees (or elbows and knees, as needed), with knees slightly spread to allow access. Her partner is on their back underneath her, with their legs lying out in front, and their face under her vulva, licking upward. This position looks a bit like a car mechanic sliding underneath a car, hence the name! Use pillows under her knees and under her partner's head for additional comfort, if desired.

Level: All levels

Degree of difficulty: 3

Pros: This position provides a great view for her partner and results in less neck strain. It allows for a different angle of access, and her partner can use their hands to stimulate additional pleasure zones on the woman's body.

Cons: It can be exhausting and even a bit frustrating for the woman to hold herself up while receiving delicious pleasure, and her partner can have trouble getting to the angles that the woman needs for ideal oral stimulation. It's hard to involve insertion (fingers or toys) in this position, it can be hard on the woman's knees, and there's always the possibility of lube dripping (which can be hot, too!).

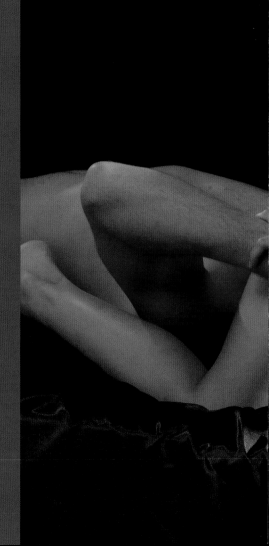

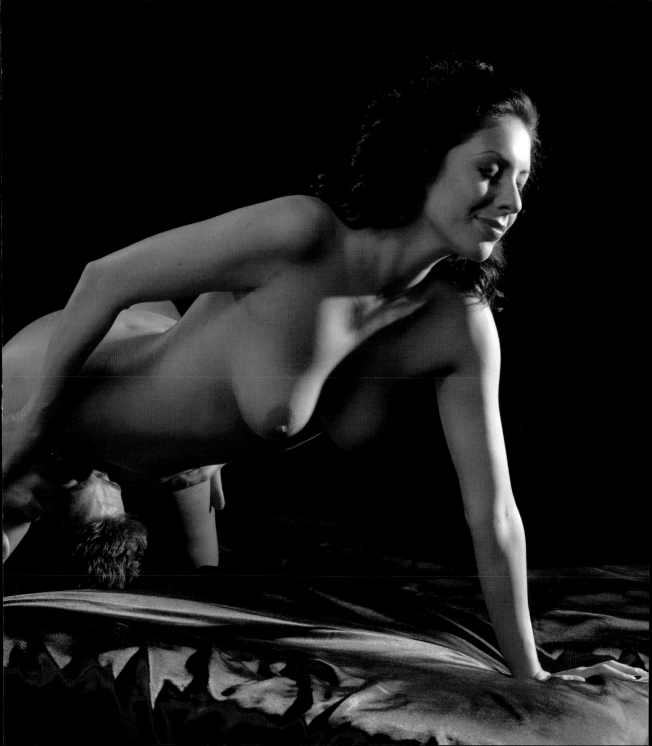

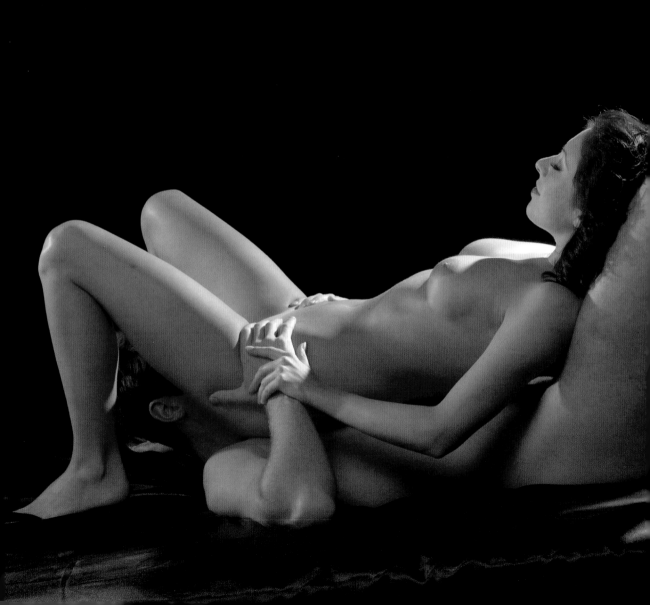

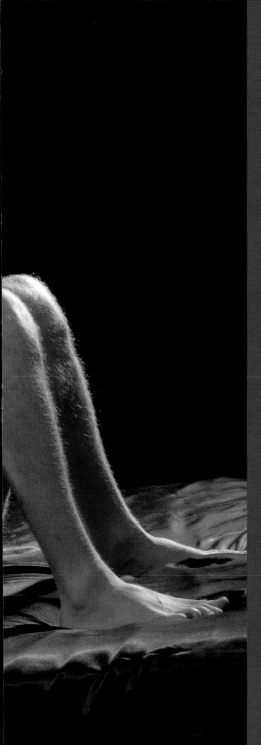

The Easy Chair

In this comfortable position, the woman uses her partner as a chair and as a backrest. The partner lies on the bed on their back, using a pillow to support their head if needed. The woman lies on top on them on her back (touching their stomach), with her feet near their head, using their bent knees as a backrest. Her vulva is at their mouth, and she can move forward or backward as needed for better access.

Level: Intermediate

Degree of difficulty: 4/5

Pros: This position allows the woman a lot more control of access to her partner, and she can move her body around to where it feels best. The position is comfortable for both partners because it doesn't require standing or flexibility, and the woman's and her partner's hands are both free to stimulate each other, and they can use toys as part of the fun.

Cons: This position requires the woman's partner to be able to comfortably bear her weight (not good for folks with knee or back problems) and for them to be similar in size. Eye contact is difficult in this position.

Pour Some Sugar on Me

This position has the woman on her knees, bent back, supporting her upper-body weight on her hands (although one hand can certainly come forward to caress her partner or to touch herself either with fingers or with a sex toy). Her partner kneels in front of her with their head in front of her vulva. The partner can also lie on their stomach with pillows to raise them to the right height, if that's more comfortable. The woman can let her head drop back, or look at her partner, or whatever works best for her. Place pillows under the woman's knees for added comfort.

Level: Intermediate

Degree of difficulty: 4/5

Pros: This position allows for eye contact between the two partners if they so decide, it can be very easy on the woman's partner's joints (especially if they choose to lie on their stomach), it provides great access to the entire vulva and breasts, and it leaves the woman with the option of having a hand free to touch herself. Power play with the woman in a dominant role can definitely be worked into this position.

Cons: Given that the woman is on her knees and bent back, it's not good for a woman with back or knee problems, and it requires a bit of flexibility, although not as much as other positions. Not the best power play position if the woman is in a submissive role. It can be hard to hold for long, and it's not easy for the woman to touch her partner's body.

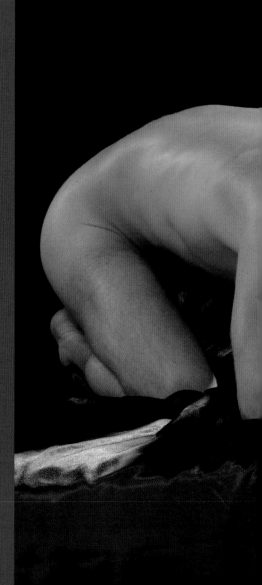

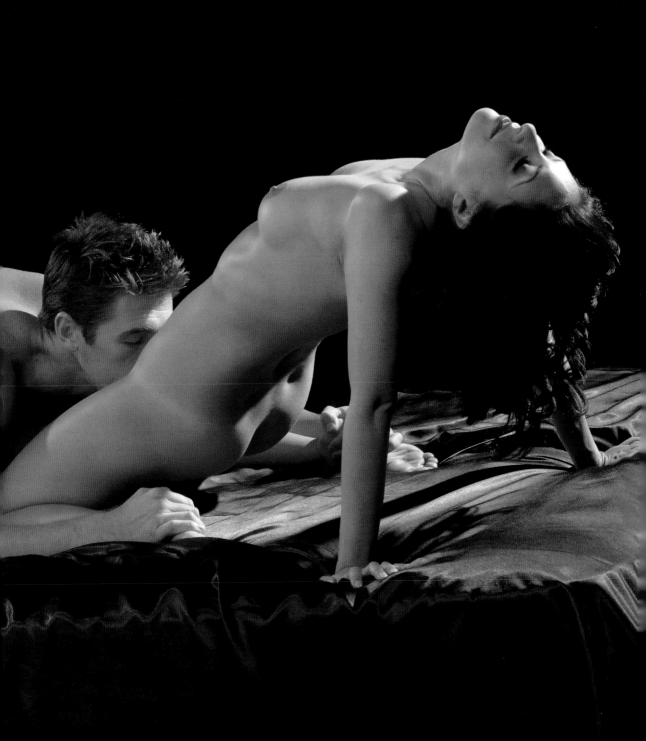

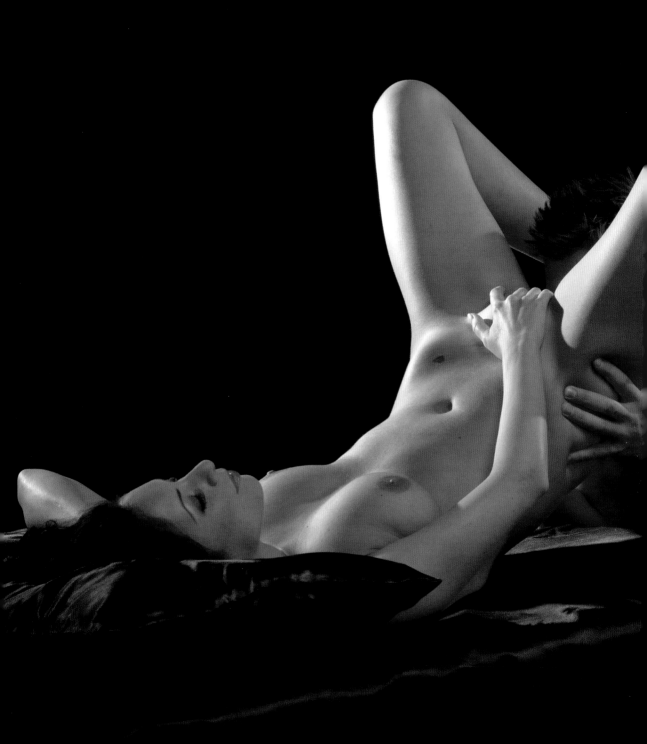

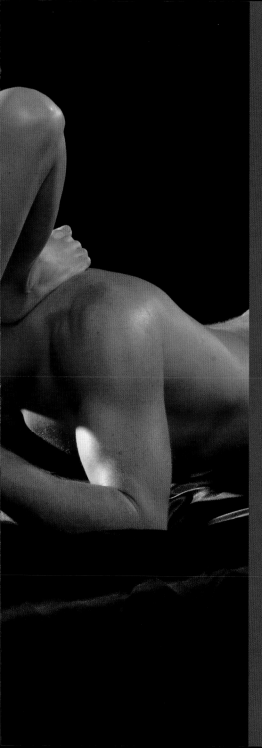

London Bridge

In this relaxing yet exciting position, the woman lies on her back in bed. Her partner lies on their stomach between her legs, and she's placed her feet on her partner's shoulders. Using her feet as leverage, she's raised her butt and pelvis off the bed (which can also be supported by pillows or her partner's arms and hands), raising her vulva to her partner's face level. She can choose to place both hands behind her head, to reach one or both down to play with/touch her partner, or to caress herself, or even to stimulate herself with a sex toy. This can be a great position for power play in which the woman is more dominant.

Level: Intermediate

Degree of difficulty: 5

Pros: In this position, the woman has complete control over access to her vulva and can change the proximity or angle in relation to her partner at any point. Her arms are free to relax, to play with herself, or to play with her partner, and this position is fairly easy on her partner's back and knees (especially with support from pillows). Because of the support of her partner, it's not too strenuous to hold, nor does it require much flexibility.

Cons: This position is not great if the woman has back or neck issues, since both are used to maintain this position. While not strenuous, it can be hard to hold for long. There is little opportunity for eye contact, and some people don't like the sensation of their feet being on someone or their partner's feet on their body.

Riding into the Night

The woman's partner lies on their back on the bed/floor/couch. The woman kneels and faces the head of the bed, with her knees resting on either side of the partner's head while straddling their face. She can place one or both hands on the wall if she needs to help support herself, and her partner's hands are free to touch, grope, grab, or slap—whatever feels best.

Level: Any

Degree of difficulty: 3

Pros: It provides a different angle of access for licking, can be coupled with some fun power play/role-play, and allows the woman to control stimulation more. Also, her partner's hands are free to roam around her body, and it definitely provides a great view of her cave of wonders.

Cons: Breathing is important for the partner and needs to be considered by the woman doing the riding. It can be hard on the woman's knees and may feel tiring to keep up for long. From the woman, it requires some semblance of balance, and this isn't a good position if the partner has feelings of claustrophobia.

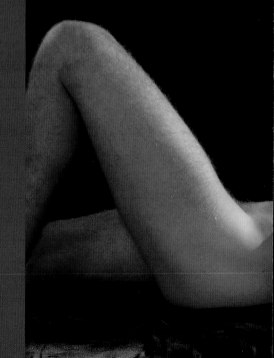

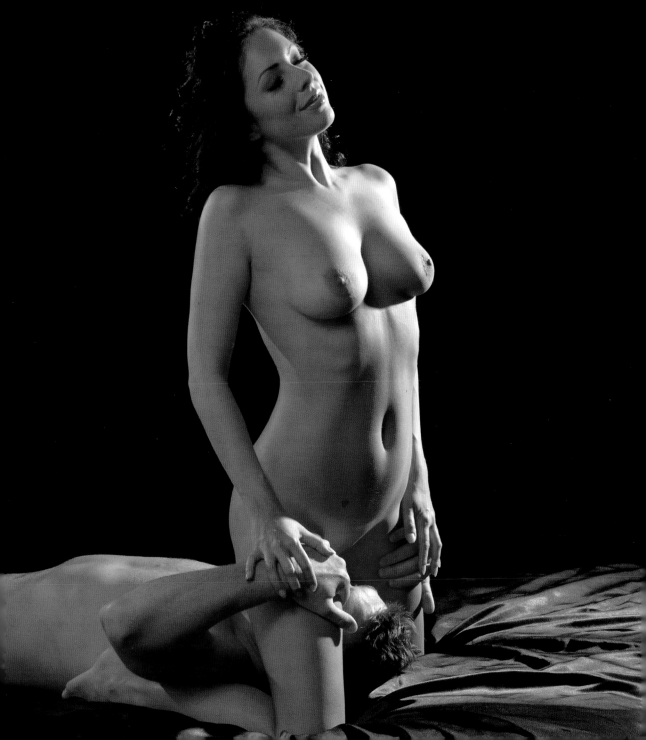

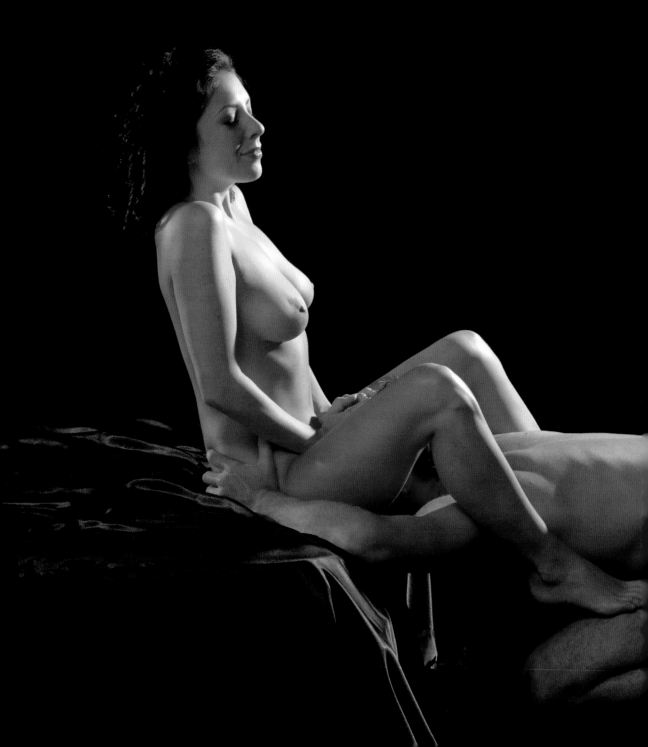

Kneeling Worship

The partner kneels on the floor at the edge of the bed facing the bed. The woman sits up straight on the edge of the bed, resting her open legs over her partner's shoulders. Her partner's head is in front of her vulva. One of her hands is wrapped in her partner's hair, holding her partner's head, the other is on the bed supporting her body. If she wants, both arms can be on the bed, or she can lie flat. Legs can be completely over the shoulders for comfort, or the feet can be braced on the shoulders, providing more access to her labia and clitoris. Add a pillow or two under her partner's knees for extra soft comfort, if wanted.

Level: Any

Degree of difficulty: 2

Pros: This allows for a great angle for access to everything and doesn't put her partner's neck at odd angles (reducing cramping). It's very comfortable for the woman, with little to no stress on any joints, and can be part of power play/role-play. It allows for changing of the legs/butt position for optimal stimulation.

Cons: This position can be rough on the partner's knees/hips (add a pillow during longer sessions), it can feel like an odd angle to some, there's little to no chance of eye contact, and it can get uncomfortable to have the legs elevated for a longer period.

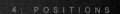

Have a Leg Up

The woman stands at the edge of the bed, facing the bed, with one leg up and bent, placing her foot on the bed, with her standing leg straight. Her partner lies on their back on the bed, with their head positioned in front of her vulva for licking. She balances herself on her partner's waist (and can also use her hands to pull her partner in closer, or push her partner away as she likes).

Level: Intermediate/Advanced

Degree of difficulty: 5

Pros: A fun and unique position, it provides a different type of access and is very comfortable for the partner, with no strain on any body parts. Both partners can get a good look at the eye candy of each other, it can be used as part of power play/role-play, and it offers good leg stretch to the standing woman (but alternate midway through this position to get equal stretching).

Cons: Requires a medium amount of balance on the woman's part, and it can be difficult to stay in for long. Sometimes there can be vaginal fluid that gets in the partner's eyes, there can be too much stress on the woman's standing leg or hip joint, and it doesn't allow for a lot of eye contact.

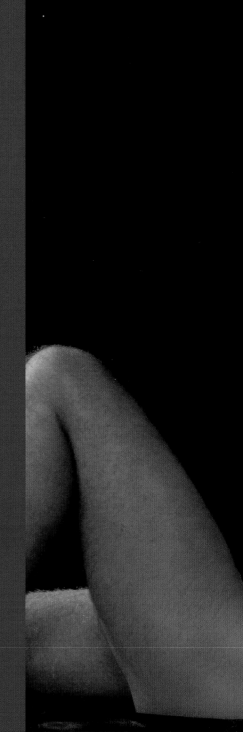

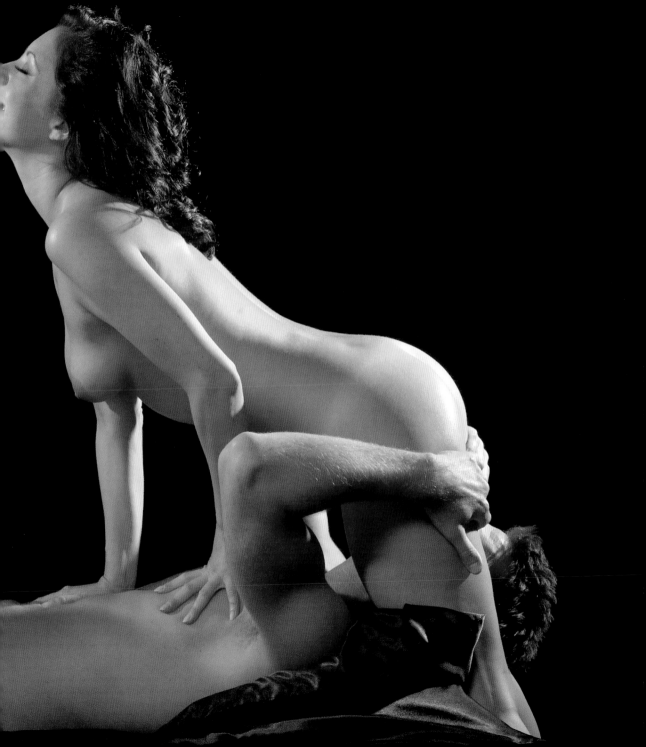

Let's Talk Toys

In the last hundred years or so, we've been lucky enough to witness the invention of a multitude of toys designed purely for sexual pleasure. From vibrators to butt plugs, dildos to cock rings, there are toys designed for pretty much every sexy activity you can think of, and probably some that haven't even occurred to you yet.

For some people, the idea of adding toys, accessories, or other exciting accoutrements can seem scary or intimidating for a variety of reasons. For others, adding a little toy action is old hat. Whether you experiment with adding toys to your sexy time play is up to you, but let's talk about some of the concerns people may have about toys for big girls and big boys.

Some people have the idea that once someone tries out a sex toy, they'll somehow magically become addicted and never again want to return to the world of human touch. I'm happy to report that there hasn't been a single real-world occurrence or any documented research of any person, regardless of gender, getting addicted to a sex toy.

First of all, sex toys, whatever type they are and whatever functions they have, don't kiss. They don't cuddle. They don't ask you what you want or communicate their needs to you. They definitely don't share in doing chores, take turns with walking the dog, or wake you up with breakfast in the morning. While they can assist you in reaching fabulous orgasms, they aren't addictive because they don't provide 99 percent of the things that a human being does.

As far as physical addiction to the sensation that the toys provide, here's the deal: you CAN get accustomed to a specific sensation, whether it's provided by a toy or by a specific person. But all you have to do to basically "re-set" your body is to take some time off from whatever that sensation is. If you feel as if you're getting used to the sensations provided by a vibrator, stop using it for a week or two or three. If you've recently changed partners, it may take a few weeks to get used to the new and different sensations provided by a new partner.

If you're considering purchasing a new sex toy for use with your partner, it's a good idea to run your sexy thoughts by them first. For many people, going shopping for the new toy together (either online or by visiting a store together) is a great way to pick out a toy that both of you are comfortable with and that both of you will like. This way, it's not just one of you picking out a toy and showing it to the other, instead you both have a vested interest in the toy, since it was one that got you both excited.

There's no shame in owning or using a sex toy (or multiple sex toys). Think of it like your kitchen supplies or your workshop. Can you roll dough by hand? Sure, but it's nice to have a rolling pin, and even a dough press to mix things up. Can you cut boards by hand and drill holes manually? Sure, but a circular saw and a power drill can make life a little more fun at times. It's nice to have lots and lots of tools to get the job done, as well as the ability to use manual labor.

Recent studies have shown that anywhere from 50 to 75 percent of women use or have used sex toys, and somewhere from 33 to 50 percent of men have done the same. Shows like *Sex and the City* have normalized sex toys for masturbation, and mainstream magazines like *Cosmo* and *Marie Claire* now regularly talk about using sex toys in relationships. While it would be hyperbolic to say that everyone's doing it, and while sex toys aren't the right fit for every individual or every couple, using sex toys is certainly acceptable today and can add a lot of fun new dimensions to your sex life, both alongside and with your partner.

So what sex toys apply to going down on your partner and having the breakfast of champions? There's a whole bevy of toys available for use by both partners during cunnilingus.

Let's start with some of the basics. You may be wondering how you can be using a vibrator while someone is giving you epic oral ministrations with their tongue. Well, luckily for us, some brilliant person came up with the design for a tongue vibrator. Yes, that's right. A tongue vibrator, a vibrator that goes around the tongue. It takes little watch batteries, so it isn't the most powerful vibrator on the market, but it provides a little extra va-va-voom and can help the cunnilingus giver with a little bit of a break for their tongue.

Speaking of giving the tongue a bit of a rest, the receiver of the oral action can step in with some of their own finger or clitoral vibrator action midcunnilingus to let the lingual lover take a quick break. While the vibrator is, well, vibrating, the giver can play with the receiver's nipples, add lots of sweet kisses, use their fingers for manual stimulation, or even take control of the toy. Just because you've brought the toy into your playtime doesn't mean that you have to keep the toy going throughout. It's OK to bring the vibe in for a little bit, and then take it out when the licker is ready to start lapping again.

Another option is to have an internal stimulation vibrator inside the vagina, buzzing away while the giver of the cunnilingus is going to town on the labia and clitoris. Many folks like the feeling of being full, and while that can be achieved by a nonvibrating dildo (as I discuss shortly), some people like the feeling of internal vibrators. The person receiving the oral loving can just let it sit, can push it in and out, or can ask their partner to actively fuck them with the vibrator while going down on them as well. Don't forget to add lube for any internal action!

If the person with the vulva likes the feeling of being full while receiving oral sex without wanting vibration, that's when the idea of using a dildo may present itself. Dildos are designed for either filling the vagina or being thrust in and out of the vagina (some dildos are also anal friendly, but only if they have a base wider than the rest of the toy). Add a little bit of water-based lubricant to keep things sliding smoothly, and either partner can help operate the dildo during oral sex.

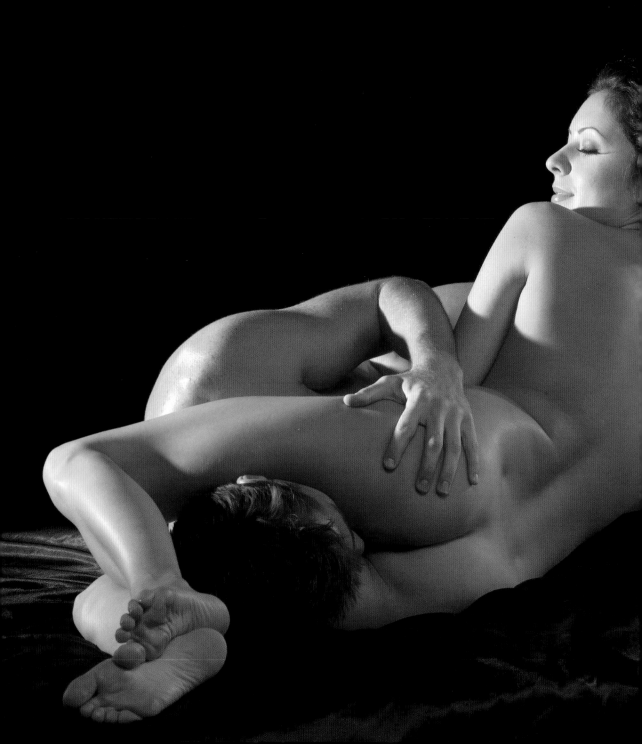

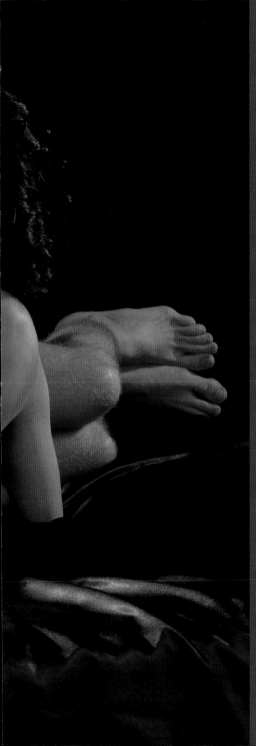

Orgasmic Earmuffs

The woman lies on her side on the bed, with her bottom leg straight out toward the bottom of the bed, and her top leg bent up, making a triangle, with the foot on her knee. She's supports herself slightly on a bent arm, looking down at her partner. Her partner lies on their side, with their head in her vulva area, resting on her thigh, with their body facing toward her head. She can also choose to bend her legs and place them more securely around her partner's ears, if she feels more comfortable that way. Feel free to use pillows both for extra comfort and to adjust angles/body positions for better stimulation.

Level: Beginner/Intermediate

Degree of difficulty: 3

Pros: This is a great position that provides comfort for both parties, since the woman's partner can rest their head on her thigh like a pillow. It's easy to maintain for a longer period, provides great access to the genital area, and doesn't require much flexibility or balance.

Cons: There isn't a lot of eye contact in this position, and it can be difficult for the woman's partner to touch, rub, and stimulate other parts of her body. It's also a more traditional, relaxed position, which may seem more run-of-the-mill to those trying to mix things up.

Up the Wall

In this position, the woman stands, with her back against the wall, her legs spread about shoulder width apart, and her arms reaching up to balance her. The woman's partner sits cross-legged between her legs, facing the wall, with both hands on her hips, pulling her vulva close to their face.

Level: Intermediate/Advanced

Degree of difficulty: 6

Pros: This is a unique and entertaining position, it's comfortable for the partner sitting on the floor, it mixes things up and is something fun to try together, it provides freedom for the partner's hands to touch and stimulate other parts of the woman's body, and eye contact can be made if desired.

Cons: This position requires a significant amount of balance on the woman's part (though she can in fact use her hands to help herself balance), and it doesn't provide access to the woman's breasts. Because of the balance required, it can cause both partners to tire more quickly, and it needs an empty wall with no furniture or window.

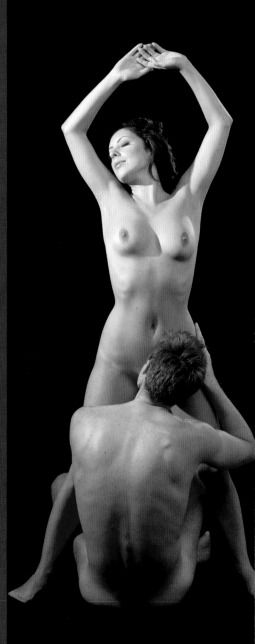

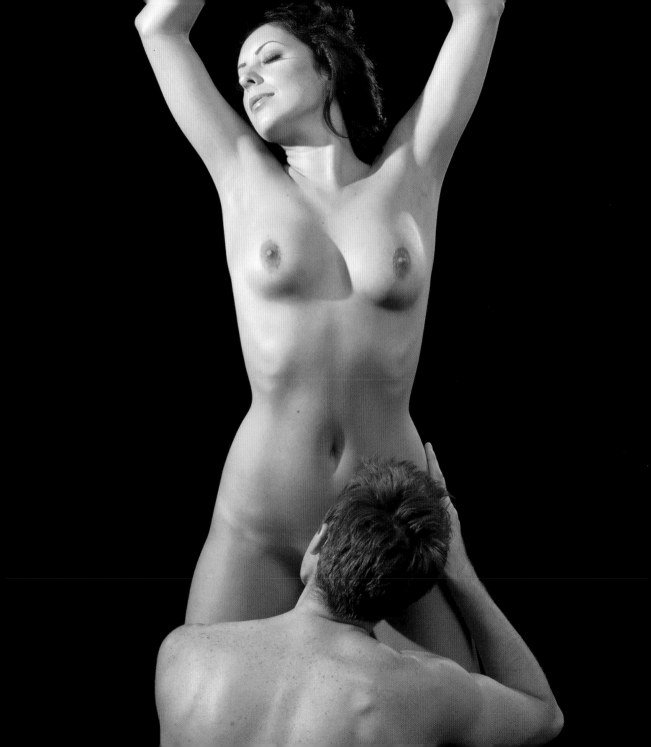

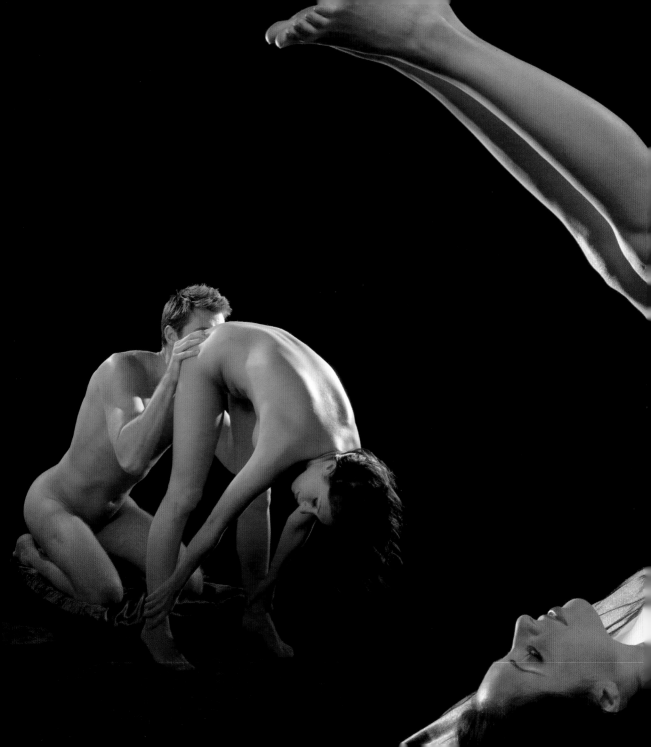

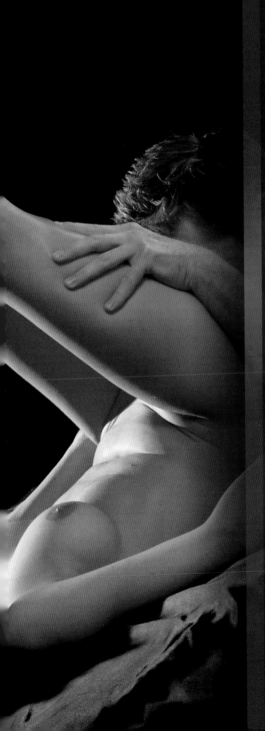

Advanced Positions

This section is advanced for a reason; these positions are a bit beyond the run-of-the-mill and would be considered advanced or even "Wow — how do they even DO that?" in some people's experiences. Do you need to be able to do these positions to have a fabulous time in the bedroom? Absolutely not. If you or your partner tend to have joint pain, bad backs, or are less than flexible, these might not be for you. If you choose to try them anyway, good on you, but please be careful. Doctors are notoriously NOT sympathetic to injuries caused by sexual mishaps.

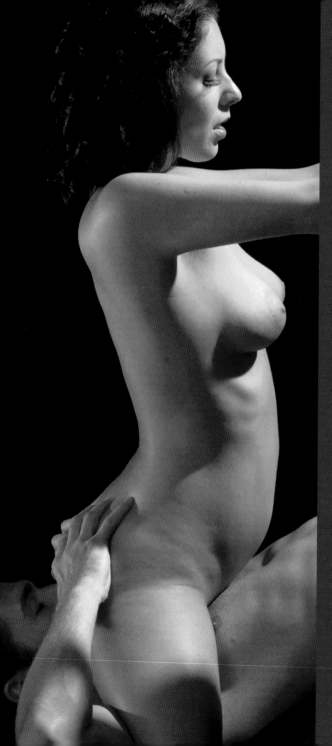

Regardless of your experience level, it's important to prepare before hopping into any of these positions. First of all, discuss the next position with your partner. Most people don't appreciate being flipped this way and that, or being turned over any which way, without knowing what the plan might be. If you're looking to mix things up in the bedroom, take a moment to browse though the following positions together. Pick out the ones you like and think you can definitely do, consider ones that look like fun, but may challenge both of your bodies (and may end up with someone falling off the bed), and realize that not every position is perfect for every couple.

Once you've made some sort of a plan and have an idea of which positions you'd like to experiment with, take a moment to get set up. If you're going to have people standing on their head or hanging off chairs, doing so on a carpet or a well-placed rug might be a good idea. If you need accessories, like a rug, chair, or a bevy of pillows, find them and place them conveniently before the clothes start flying. That way, when you're in the middle of position A and want to switch to position B, there won't need to be a pause for collecting accessories.

Also keep in mind that if a position requires flexibility, it might be worth warming up your limbs (and those of your partner). It doesn't have to be a session at the ballet barre; stretch out different body parts as you make out, kiss

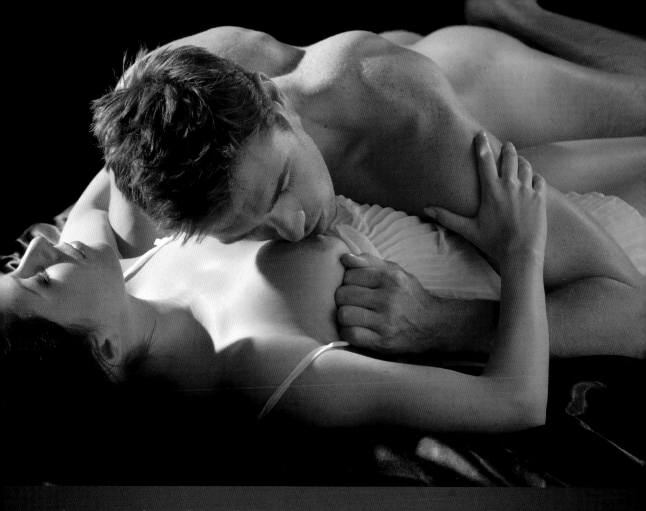

various areas, and move down to dining at the Y. Making out can be a great way to try different positions as well and get your various body parts ready for a raucous workout.

Last but not least, the point of trying new positions is to mix things up and have fun. Some of these positions might work admirably for you and your partner, and go in your repertoire to do over and over. Others might not be a success, and that's OK, too. Sex is a journey of experimentation and having pleasure; laughter is just as pleasurable as an orgasm, and if it didn't work for you, mark that position off and head to the next one. Keep in mind that sex is fun, and laughter is beneficial, and a good time should be had by all!

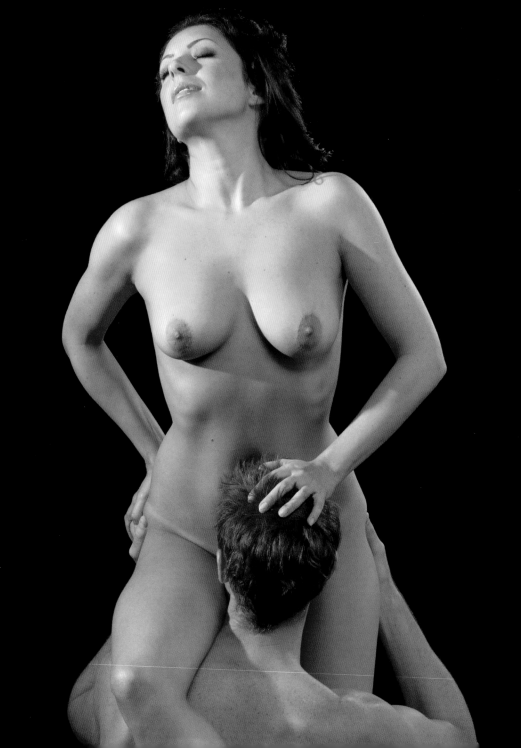

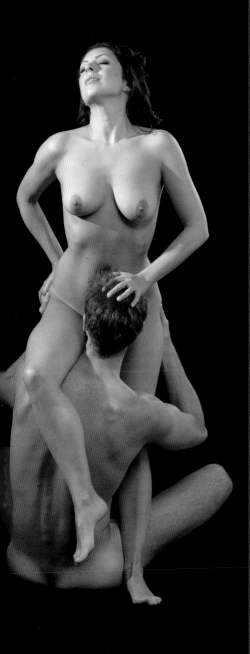

Leg Over Easy

The woman's partner sits on the ground with legs crossed, back as straight as possible. Facing her partner, the woman stands, with one leg over her partner's back, allowing her partner complete access to her vulva. Her hands can be used to brace herself on the wall, or her hands can be placed on her partner's shoulders, or they can be holding on to her partner's head (or any combination thereof).

Level: Advanced

Degree of difficulty: 7

Pros: It's a fairly easy and laid-back position for the woman's partner, it doesn't require too much flexibility, it does offer a different angle of access to the genitals, it can be a lot of fun and mixes things up, and it can be used in a woman-dominant power play setting.

Cons: This position requires a high level of balance for the woman, her partner doesn't have access to her breasts or upper body for caressing, it can get uncomfortable/tiring more quickly than certain other positions, and it requires an empty wall or excellent balance.

Lengthy Legs

In this position, the woman lies on her back, with her head on a pillow. Her legs are straight, but bent at the hips, as if she's been folded in half. One of her hands (or both, if she prefers), can hold her legs up, bringing them close to her, or if she has the ab strength, she can just hold them up without using hands. Her partner lies on their side at an angle to her, almost forming an L-shape along her body, able to lick and stimulate her vulva through her raised legs.

Level: Advanced

Degree of difficulty: 7

Pros: Because this position involves both partners lying down, there's not a high need for balance for either person. It doesn't require much flexibility from the partner, and with the woman holding her legs (or using a rope/cloth), it can be held for longer periods without tying. The position leaves her partner's hands free to play with her and stimulate her, as well as provides a fun and unique angle from which to approach the vulva.

Cons: This position doesn't allow for much eye contact, it can be a position that may make climax difficult for certain people, it can be hard to hold for long, it requires a pillow and a comfortable surface to lie on, and the woman must be flexible enough to bend into it.

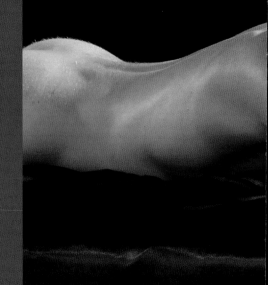

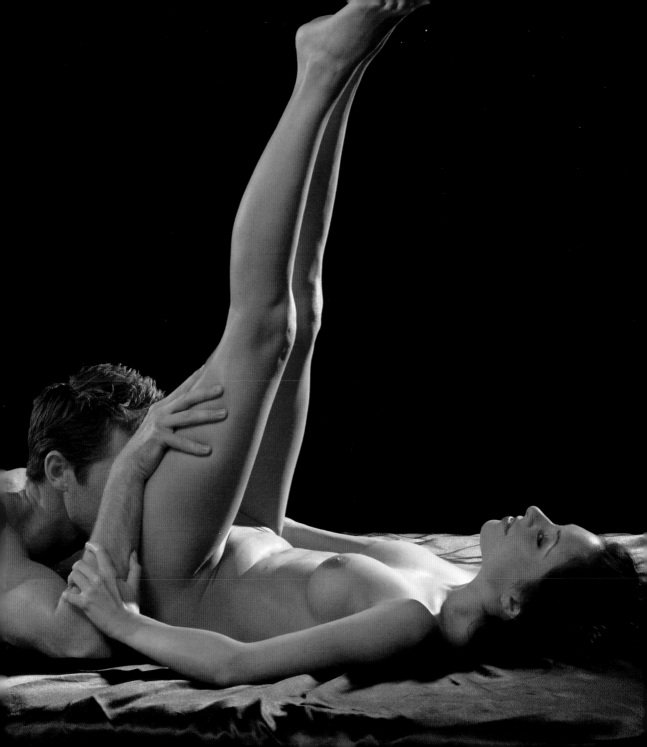

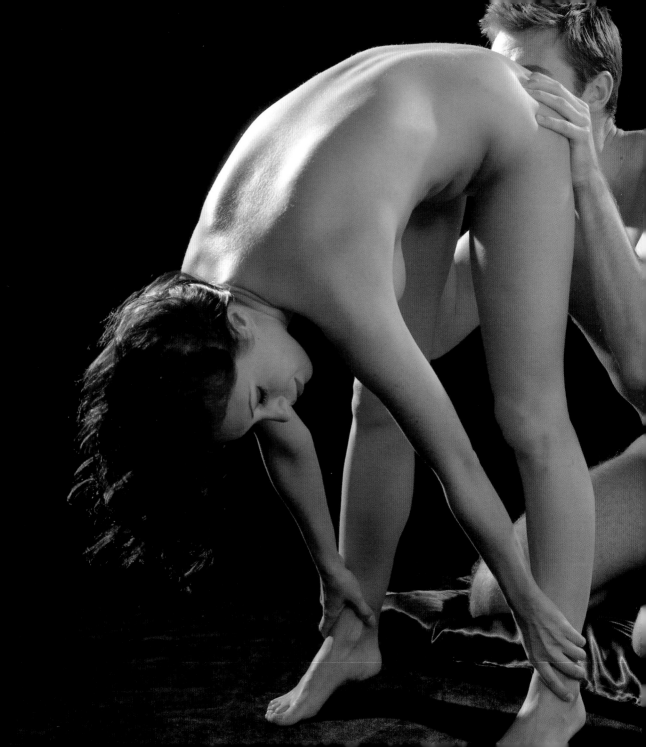

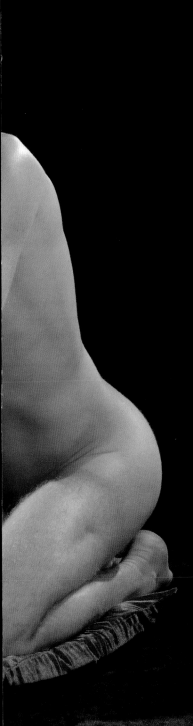

Forward Fold

The woman stands, bent over forward, with her hands on her ankles, legs spread about shoulder width apart. Her partner kneels behind her, holding her hips on the side or front, with their face near her vulva from the rear. For added comfort, place a pillow under the partner's knees.

Level: Advanced

Degree of difficulty: 8

Pros: This is a unique position that adds an element of hot anonymous sex because there's no face-to-face contact, doesn't require much flexibility or balance by the partner, can be done without any walls/beds/furniture, and can be done quickly as part of a series of positions without much difficulty in moving around.

Cons: This position requires a great deal of balance and flexibility on the woman's part, it doesn't provide a lot of access to the vulva, the angle makes it difficult for many people to orgasm, the rush of blood to the head can be uncomfortable to many people, and there's no eye contact.

Temple of the Goddess

The woman kneels (she can place a pillow underneath her knees for additional comfort), with her knees spread, leaning back, supporting herself with at least one hand. With her other hand, she can be supporting her weight, playing with herself (with or without a vibrator), or grasping her partner's hair. Her partner kneels in front of her (place a pillow under their knees if they'd like to be more comfortable), with their head almost touching the bed as their mouth rests in front of her vulva for licking and sucking. Another variation is to have her partner on their back, sliding their head in between her legs, as shown in this image.

Level: Advanced

Degree of difficulty: 8

Pros: This is a fun position that can involve power play or role-play of pussy/Goddess worship, and it's comfortable in a bed and provides a new angle of access to her vulva. Her partner doesn't need much balance or much flexibility, can use both hands all over her body, and can make eye contact by looking up at her.

Cons: It requires a good bit of flexibility and balance on the woman's part, especially if she plans to hold herself in this position for any period of time. It can be rough on the knees and hip joints of both partners, especially when they're on a hard surface or not using pillows.

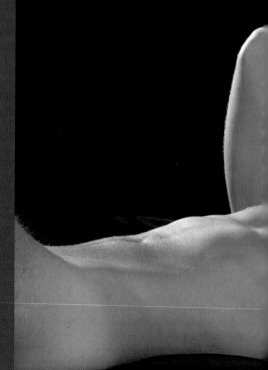

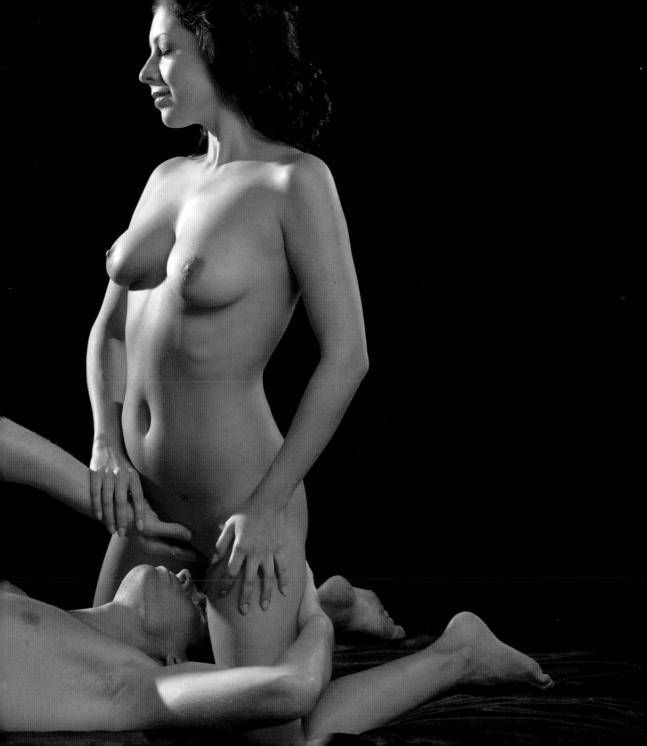

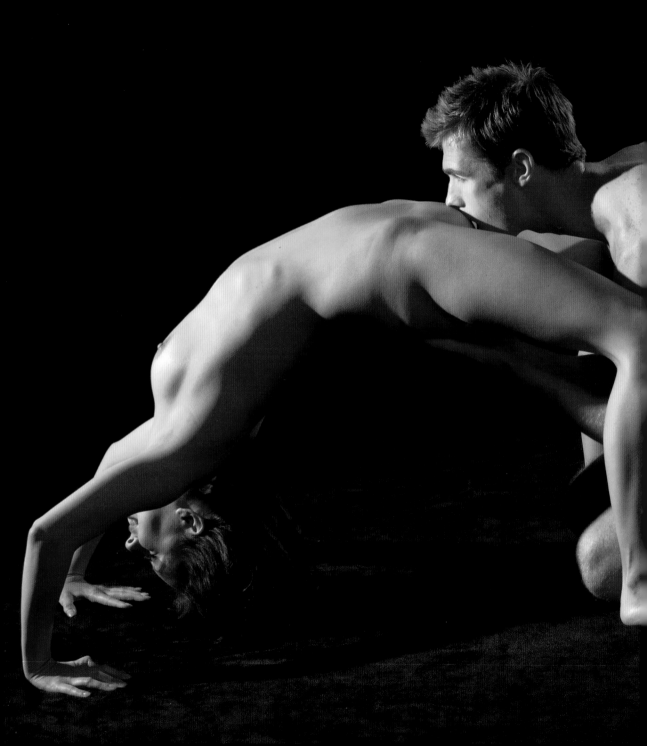

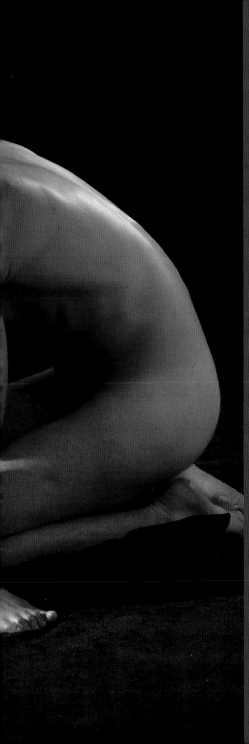

Bending Bridges

The woman is bent back in a bridge pose (which in yoga is frequently known as Wagon Pose). Her partner kneels in front of her by her legs (place a pillow underneath their knees for additional comfort), with their face near/directly in front of her vulva and their hands reaching around to clasp her butt. It's highly recommended to do this position on a softer surface for at least the first few times to avoid injury, and pre–sexy time stretching (or involving stretching as part of foreplay) might be an excellent idea.

Level: Advanced

Degree of difficulty: 10

Pros: This is definitely one of those positions that will wow everyone involved (and anyone who is told about it): it provides an entirely new angle of access to the woman's genitals, it doesn't require much flexibility or balance from her partner, and it's a form of exercise on top of the normal calorie burning from sex.

Cons: One of the hardest positions to sustain while receiving pleasure, it requires both flexibility and balance on the woman's part, and those who have yoga experience will have an easier time. No eye contact is possible, and her partner's hands do not have access to much, especially if they're helping stabilize her.

All-Over-the-Body Toys

While it's not everyone's cup of tea, some people love some butt action. If you or your partner enjoy anal stimulation, inserting an anal vibrating dildo, anal beads, or a butt plug (vibrating or not) before going down can provide a continued sensation in that area. Keep in mind that EITHER partner (or both partners!) can enjoy anal stimulation during the act of oral sex, and it can help to pleasure the giver while they're concentrating on vulvar loving. Remember that you ALWAYS need to use lubricant when working with the anus, and that anything you place in the butt needs to have a flanged base, a base wider than the rest of the toy. Clitoral vibrators and dildos without a base don't ever belong in the butt. Warm up the anus a bit before placing anything in it, and remember, if you touch the butt, wash your hands or change gloves before touching the vulva, as you can transfer unfriendly bacteria and cause infections in the vulva and vagina.

Which butt toy is right for you? Butt beads are meant to be placed in one at a time and can be gently pulled out during or right around the time of orgasm. An anal dildo is meant more to go in and out (either partner can operate this), while a butt plug (vibrating or not) is meant to be worked in, and then left in place during whatever activity is taking place. Check out the different sizes, shapes, and options, and find the one (or ones) that look most appealing to you and your partner.

Other fun toys can make oral sex even a bit more orgasmic. One item that's certainly an accessory in the bedroom (or anywhere) that can get more senses tingling is the blindfold! Whether you go out and buy a fancy blindfold to match your boudoir or you just pick up a random hanky lying around, blindfolding the receiver of the oral is fun. This increases all of the other sensations, and so touches will feel more intense, and you can play to other senses with food, sexy and sensual music, and scented candles or incense. This can ramp up the experience for the person wearing the blindfold, and if they don't like the feeling, they can always remove it easily and quickly.

Another above-the-belt sex toy is nipple clamps. While these might seem intense and scary to some people, nipple clamps can go from mild to wild. They're perfect for any nipples, regardless of what size the areolas are, what the person's gender is, or whether they're pierced. Nipple clamps can include tweezer clamps, alligator clamps, and clover clamps. I'd recommend newbies start with tweezer clamps, as they're easily adjustable and don't get too tight. If that doesn't provide enough sensation for you or your partner, feel free to step up to alligator clamps, or even clover clamps. If you're not ready to invest in nipple clamps to start with, wooden clothespins provide an admirable substitute and can be loosened by placing rubber bands around the tips. Just remember to start easy and work your way up, and not to leave nipple clamps or clothespins on for more than about twenty minutes. They usually hurt a bit coming off as well, so keep that in mind. If all of this sounds like too much, superlightweight vibrating nipple clamps are available, and you can even find nipple pumps that provide lots of fun sensation, but without any amount of "ow!"

It can be fun to add a little kink to your playtime as well. Bondage can go a long way to keeping the spice in your sex life. Be careful about using handcuffs (real or play ones), since metal pressing against wrists can cause nerve damage in some folks. But wrist and ankle restraints can be a fun, simple, and comfortable way to immobilize either the giver or receiver as you take turns giving each other all types of naughty pleasure. You can just bind your lover's cuffs, or you can use the nylon-webbing under-bed systems designed for restraining your partner without having to do hard-core construction in the bedroom. Another thing you can experiment with are scarves or ties, but please remember these tend to get tighter and tighter as they're pulled on (as do panty hose or nylons!), so it's worth having a pair of medical shears or safety scissors in case any knots or ties accidentally get too tight. If anyone's hands get cold or turn blue, make sure to take the bondage off right away. Start slow and work your way up; it's always more fun to add more spice than to scare your lover off by showing up with an entire working dungeon without discussing it first!

Sensation play in combination with blindfolds and/or bondage can be superdelightful for either or both of you. Feather ticklers can feel fabulous, and even household items like basting brushes, toothpicks, hairbrushes, loofahs, and so on provide different and exciting sensations as they're gently moved over your lover's skin. If they're blindfolded, you can ask them to guess what you're using on them, and if they're tied up, you can caringly torment and tickle them until they can't take it anymore. As with any and all power play, if the word "no" doesn't mean no anymore (like "Oh no, no, that feels so intense, I just can't take it any more" . . . when they really want you to keep going), you need to decide on a new word to mean no, like red, or halt, or cantaloupe. This is also true of role-plays that involve power dynamics, as well as bondage, gagging, or any play that might need a word to indicate an ALL PLAY STOPS NOW type of limit. Remember to discuss new directions of sexy time, toys, and so forth with your partner instead of just springing new things on them, and you're sure to have a much more exciting time together!

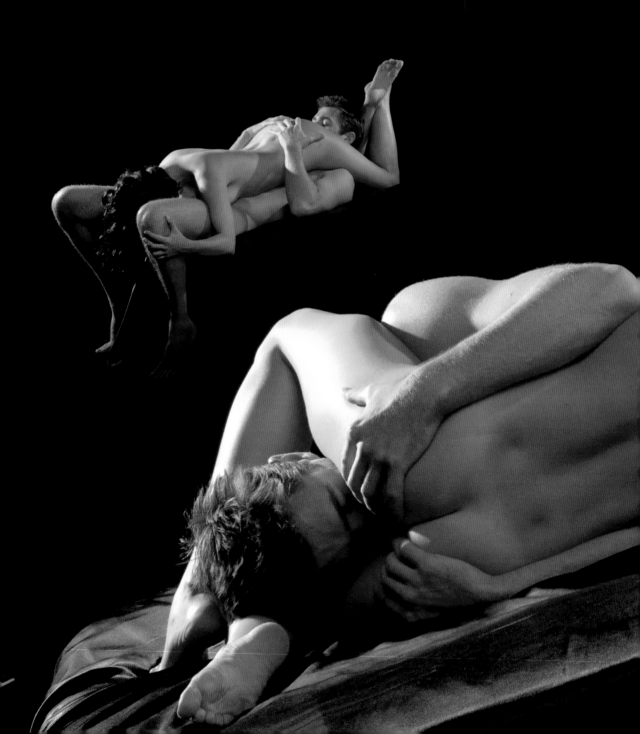

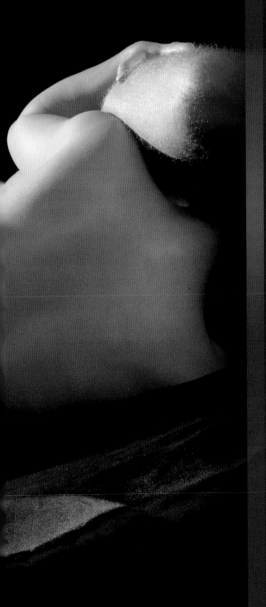

68 and 69 Positions

***These positions allow both partners to enjoy receiving stimulation from each other* . . .** at the same time. Most of the following positions are designed so that both parties get oral sex simultaneously, but it's also possible for one person to enjoy oral stimulation from their partner, while the other receives a hand job or gets fingered. Also, both partners can provide manual stimulation to their partner simultaneously, either as a break from oral sex (to let your tongue/lips/mouth/jaw) recover a bit, or as a fun event in and of itself.

It's important to take a moment to talk about the oft-worshipped concept of both partners magically orgasming at the same time. CAN this happen? Yes, I suppose it can. Does it happen regularly? No, it doesn't. First of all, many people find it difficult to concentrate on enjoying their own sensations and feelings while they're also concentrating on providing delectable sensations and pleasure to a partner. This doesn't mean that both of you cannot enjoy providing each other pleasure at the same time, it just means that making it to orgasm (assuming that's your goal) might be a bit more difficult for one or both of you.

Also, the likelihood that two different people (regardless of their genders) will take EXACTLY the same amount of time to reach climax is pretty slim. Again, CAN it happen? Sure. Is it likely to happen? Not really, and definitely not every time. For some reason, we've been fed this myth that having orgasms at the EXACT SAME TIME is somehow proof of us being with the right partner, having a special connection, and so forth. Baloney! Plus, if you both happen to orgasm at the same time, you won't get to enjoy watching your partner's face and hearing their yummy noises as they crash through the waves of their orgasm. So basically, if the two of you happen to have simultaneous orgasms — mazel tov! It can and does happen. But if you and your partner never blast off at the exact same time, it means absolutely nothing about your connection, your chemistry, or your relationship. It just means that you have

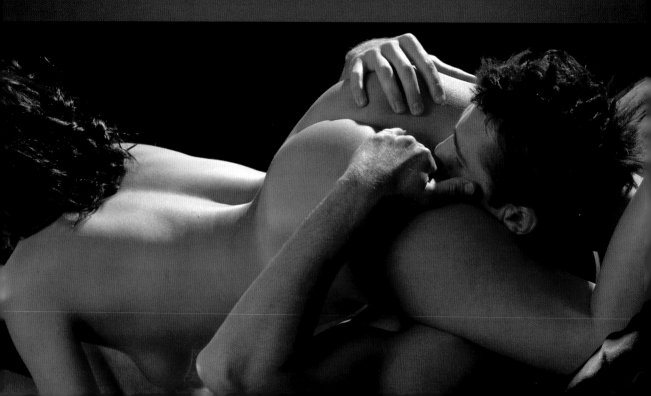

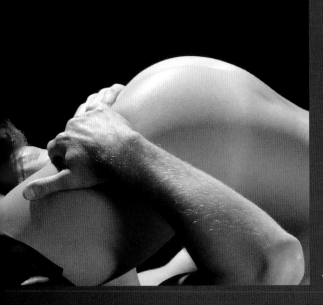

orgasm/bite down phase, you may want to remove your mouth from your partner's genital region and continue stimulating with your fingers, hands, or a toy while you enjoy the sensations. Then, once you're back in control of your various muscles and are no longer going to inadvertently cause your partner harm, you can go back to going down.

For some people, dual stimulation/69 positions can feel more intimate, like both partners are mutually involved in pleasure, or they may just like trying something new and different. For other people, they may try one of the following positions and have more of a "meh" type reaction, or find that they have trouble concentrating on giving AND receiving pleasure at the same time. Still others may enjoy these types of positions, but not absolutely love them, and will then use them as parts of foreplay, afterplay, or transitions. All of these reactions are absolutely valid, and whether you're 100 percent behind 68 and 69, or you feel that it falls a little flat for you, you're enjoying your sexual adventure, and THAT is what matters.

different things that get you going, and that it takes different amounts of time for you to get there. Enjoy figuring those things out together!

Another point to talk about in regard to dual oral sex action is keeping your head . . . and I'm not talking about the head that you're giving or getting. Oftentimes, when someone orgasms, they may clench their fingers or bite down. If you're just hanging out, enjoying some awesome oral, no big deal—no harm, no foul. But if you tend to be a jaw clencher, and you have someone's delicate naughty bits in your mouth, you need to be a bit more cognizant of what's going on. If you're about to hit the

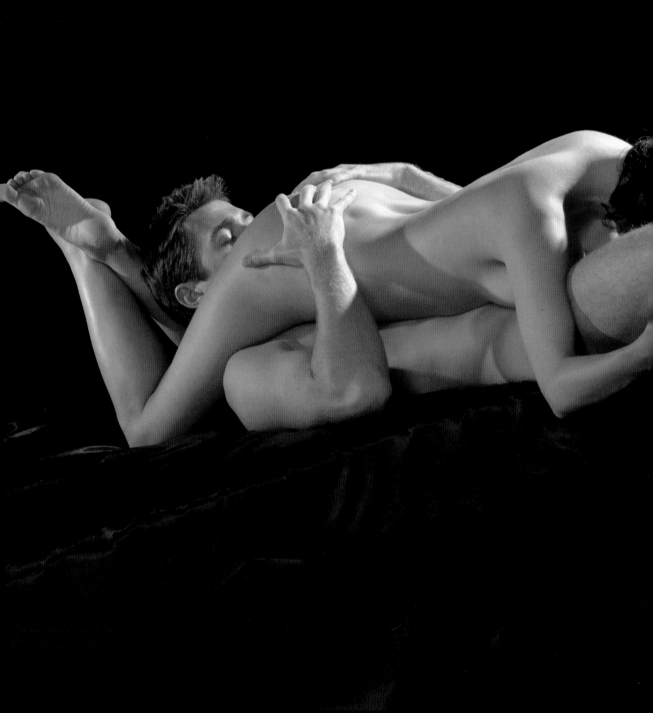

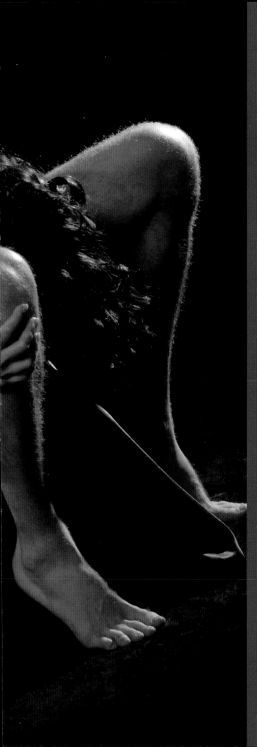

Traditional 69

In this position, the woman's partner lies on the bed, on their back, with their head placed on one or more pillows. The woman has her legs spread on either side of their shoulders (usually on her knees), while facing her partner's body, with her head near her partner's crotch. Both the woman and her partner should be licking/ sucking/stimulating each other. Pillows can be placed below her knees for additional comfort, and below her partner's back and butt to provide a better angle.

Level: **All levels**

Degree of difficulty: **3**

Pros: Tried and true, this is a fairly comfortable and relaxing position for the partner, requiring no flexibility or balance on their behalf. It doesn't need much balance or flexibility from the woman, it is fairly comfortable and can be sustained for a longer period, and it can have some power play going on.

Cons: Like most 69 style positions, there isn't a lot of opportunity for eye contact in this position, and it's not made for a woman who has bad knees. Some women cannot climax in this position, and there isn't a lot of access to other fun and exciting parts of the body of either participant.

Sliding Spoons

Here the woman lies on her side with her bottom leg straight out, and her top leg bent up with foot on knee, creating a triangle of sorts with the top leg. Her partner lies on their side, facing her, with their head between her legs, and their own legs (and genitals) near her face for possible 69 action. Both either rest their heads on the arms closest to the bed/floor/couch or use the lower arm to prop up their heads for better angles. Pillows can be used to support either person's head for additional comfort and can be used under other parts of the body to create better angles for stimulation.

Level: All levels

Degree of difficulty: 2

Pros: Since both parties are lying down, it's a comfortable position that can be held for a long period. It doesn't put pressure on the knees or the lower back, nor does it require flexibility or balance from either participant. It allows for each partner's top arm to reach over to caress, fondle, and otherwise stimulate additional spots on their partner's body.

Cons: This position doesn't allow for much eye contact between partners (although it can be done), many people (of all genders) may find it difficult to reach orgasm while lying on their side, it may seem a bit plain after a while, and the lower arms can fall asleep if in this position for too long.

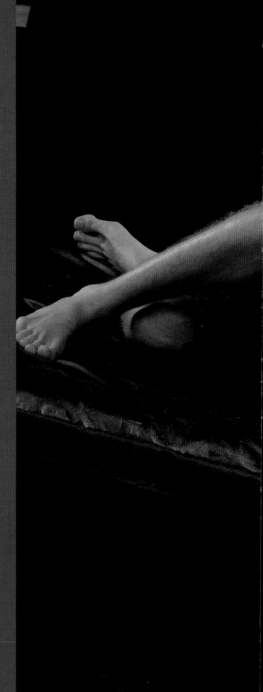

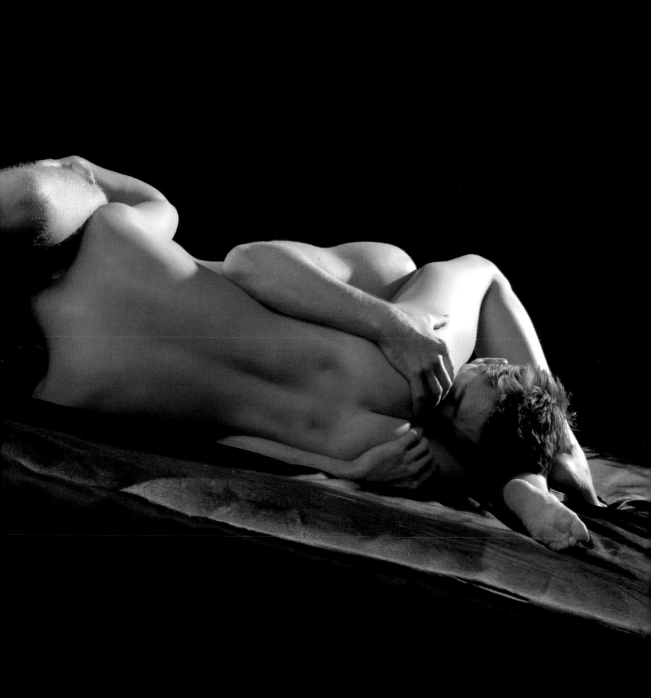

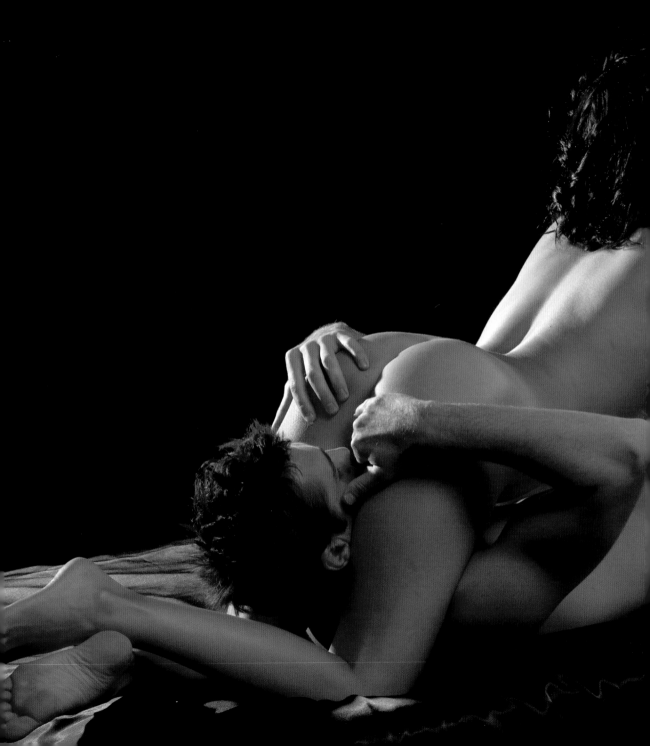

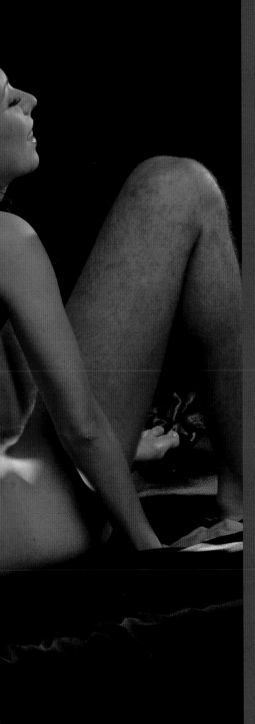

Sweet Handiwork

This position has the woman's partner lying on the bed, on their back, with their head resting on one or more pillows. The woman has her legs spread on either side of her partner's shoulders (usually in a kneeling position), facing her partner's body, with her head near her partner's knees. She's supporting herself with one of her arms, and using her hand and other arm to stimulate her partner. Her partner is licking/sucking/stimulating her vulva while she's stimulating them with her hand and fingers. Her partner can also choose to manually stimulate the woman, making this into a hot mutual masturbation position.

Level: **All levels**

Degree of difficulty: **3**

Pros: A bit of a twist on the traditional 69 position, this allows the woman to concentrate a little bit more on receiving oral sex while still giving her an opportunity to stimulate her partner. It doesn't require any flexibility or much balance on the part of either partner, and it's not hard on the partner's knees, hips, or back. The partner can use their free hands to reach up, down, and around to stimulate other parts of the woman's body.

Cons: This position can be hard on the woman's knees (place pillows underneath her knees for additional comfort), it doesn't provide an easy way to share eye contact, it may be difficult for the woman to support herself for longer periods, and it may seem too simple for couples who are into more advanced positions.

Safer Sex

Another myth often thrown around is that you can't transmit sexually transmitted infections through either giving or receiving cunnilingus. While it IS true that oral sex is often a less risky activity than some other options, STIs CAN in fact be transmitted via oral-vulvar (and oral-penile and oral-anal) stimulation.

How can you protect yourself? First of all, chat up your partner. Find out the last time they got tested was, and WHAT STIs they were tested for — lots of doctors don't run a full panel, so it's good to know which ones were tested for. Make sure you share your own testing history with your partner; it takes two to tango, or transmit, as the case may be.

Second, talk about whether either of you wants to use a barrier like a dam, a condom cut in half, a glove, and so forth. If ONE of you wants to use a barrier, then you both should, so that the person who wants it feels that their sexual health wishes are being respected.

What's a dam? It's a very thin square or rectangle of latex. You put lube on the area that you'll be licking, place the dam on top of it, and lick away! The problem with dams is that they tend to be hard to find, expensive, and not great for those with latex sensitivities.

One solution? Take an unrolled condom and cut it in half, from tip to the base (lengthwise). Voila — you have a mini-dam, and you can even use flavored condoms, lubricated or not, or nonlatex condoms. You can find flavored condoms at most groceries, drugstores, and sex toy/adult shops. Keep in mind that some flavored lubricants may contain glycerin, so check on that if either you or your partner has a glycerin sensitivity. Stay away from using spermicidal condoms for oral action; they tend to taste nasty.

Another great trick is to take a glove (latex, nitrile, or vinyl), cut off the four finger spaces, and slice along the NON-thumb side. Open in, and now you have a dam with a little finger hole for you to stimulate inside as well. Ta-da! Gloves are cheap en masse, and you can find them at the grocery, drugstore, or even a beauty supply shop. Just remember that if you or your partner has a latex allergy, stick with either the nitrile or vinyl options. Gloves can come in various colors, so feel free to match them to your outfit, your bedroom decor, or anything that comes to mind.

Yet one more supereasy-to-make alternative is to use cling wrap, or plastic wrap, from the kitchen. The nice thing is that most people already have this on hand, it comes in lots of pretty colors, and you can actually see what's beneath the wrap and enjoy what you're licking. All plastic wrap is latex free, so it's preferable for use, regardless of whether either of you have a latex allergy.

You can cut up gloves in order to create a barrier or you can just use them as is. Gloves are awesome for many reasons, not only because they protect against STIs that can be transmitted person to person by vaginal fluid on hands. If the person doing the fingering/fucking/manual stimulating has hang nails, or long nails, or sharp nails, using gloves can help prevent the person being pleasured from getting small cuts and tears in and around their vagina. Also, vaginal fluid tends to be slightly acidic, so if you're spending time playing around there, gloves can protect hands from feeling a slight stinging sensation in small cuts and rough patches. If the person doing the work has long nails, you can pop half a cotton ball into the tip of each finger in the glove before putting it on, and they're no longer a vaginal hazard. Not only that, but gloves can help lubricant (both natural and store bought) last longer. Since humans are water based, our bodies tend to absorb water-based lubrication (including the type that bodies produce) at a quicker rate than a gloved surface. Finally, wearing gloves makes for superquick cleanup, or moving to the next sexual activity, or cuddling. They come in various materials and colors, so feel free to experiment.

What are some ways to make the use of barriers feel better and sexier? Using lubricant between the barrier and the vulva can help transmit the sensations being provided. Think of it as a safer-sex sandwich — vulva, lube, barrier, tongue. You can read more in the lubricants section. Also, you can have the person receiving oral sex hold the barrier to help be more involved. There are even fancy dam-holder harnesses, or the receiver can wear a garter belt and use the straps/clips to hold the barrier in place, making for hands-free oral action. And if the dam or barrier is pulled tightly, it transmits humming VERY well, and that can feel amazing for the person getting the oral worship.

Do you HAVE to use dams or barriers? Certainly not — you don't HAVE to do anything. But it's important to be educated on safer sex and sexual health, and it's important to make sure that your partner is as well. STIs like herpes, chlamydia, and gonorrhea can all be transmitted through cunnilingus, and sometimes, bacterial infections and allergic reactions can be triggered if the person going down has recently smoked or used other chemicals orally. If you and your partner have agreed to be monogamous, and have both been recently tested for a full panel of STIs at a clinic or doctor's office, that's a different conversation to have than if you're having a hot one-night stand, or if you or your partner tends to have multiple partners. Knowledge is power; use knowledge to make the best decisions for yourself.

Though not TECHNICALLY part of the safer-sex discussion, don't forget that vulvas and vaginas are often sensitive to sugar- and glucose-based products. This means that you should probably keep whipped cream, chocolate syrup, Popsicles, lollipops, and the like far away from any action below the belt, or else you or your oh-so-pleasure partner might end up with a totally uninvited yeast infection. "Gimme some sugar" = good. "Give the vagina some sugar" = bad.

A Roll in the Hay

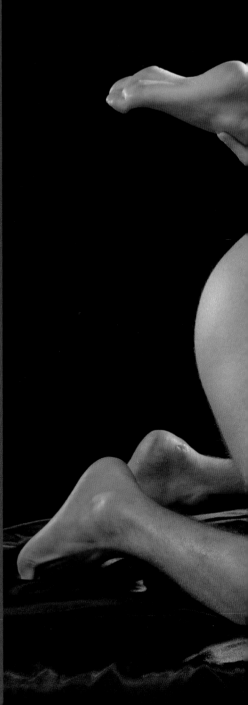

Here the woman lies on her back on the bed, with her legs open slightly (can be bent if needed), folded back toward her body, her hands holding her ankles. Her partner kneels by her head (a knee on each side of her head), and leans between her open legs, bending forward to lick, suck, and stimulate her while supporting themselves on the bed with hands on either side of her hips. Use pillows under her back or butt to help get her to the best angle, and place pillows under her partner's knees for added comfort, if desired.

Level: Intermediate

Degree of difficulty: 5

Pros: A new take on the more traditional 69 position, the open legs provide a lot more access to the woman's vulva, requiring only low flexibility on the woman's part and none from her partner. It's easy on the woman's back and knees, and she can control the angle of access to her genitals better by opening/closing and bending/straightening her legs.

Cons: It can be harder on the partner's knees and requires that her partner have some balance, and that she have at least some flexibility. Like most 69 positions, there's not a lot of opportunity for eye contact, and because everyone's hands are busy holding themselves up or holding their legs, it's difficult to stimulate each other.

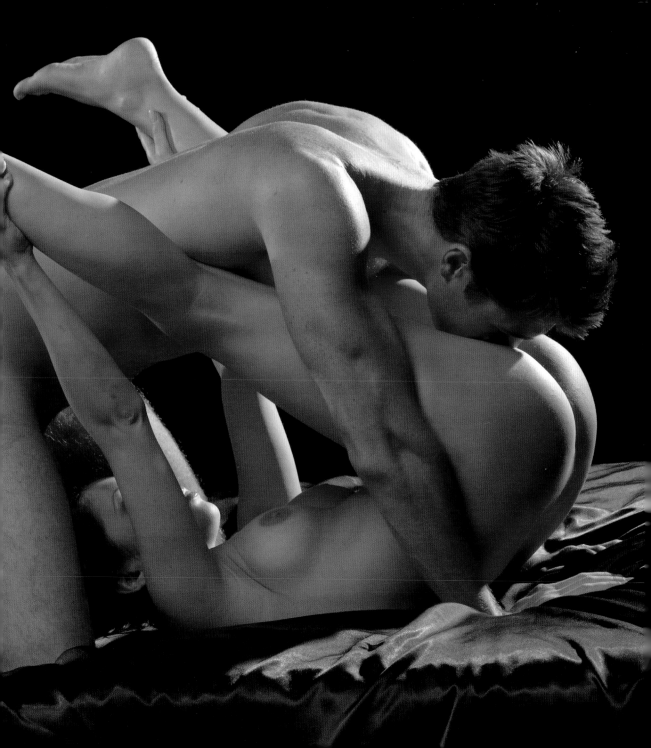

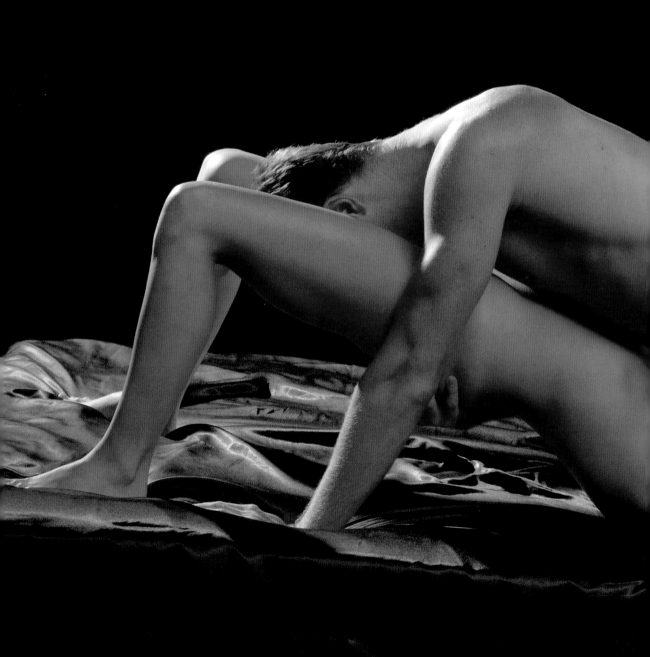

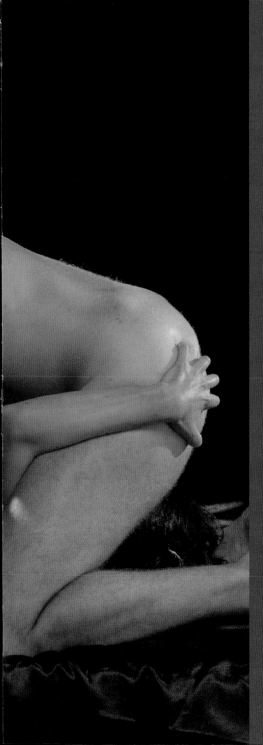

Minding the Gap

In this position that's a slight tweak on the usual 69 position of having the woman on the bottom and her partner on top, the woman lifts her hips and pelvis up to her partner's mouth, allowing them more access to her genitals, providing a stretch for her, and far less pressure on her partner's back. The supernice thing about this position is that the woman can always place her hips down for a break while staying in this general position, and just hoist them up again if it feels better for her.

Level: Intermediate

Degree of difficulty: 6

Pros: This position allows the woman a lot more control of access to her genitals, it provides a way to do this more traditional position with less strain on her partner's back, it can be supported by pillows if she's having trouble holding it, and her partner can use their hands to help support her/bring her body closer to them.

Cons: This position is not great if the woman has back or knee issues, it allows for little eye contact/cuddling, it can be exhausting if held for long, and it doesn't allow the woman much control over how much of her partner's genitals are in her mouth or how close they are to her face.

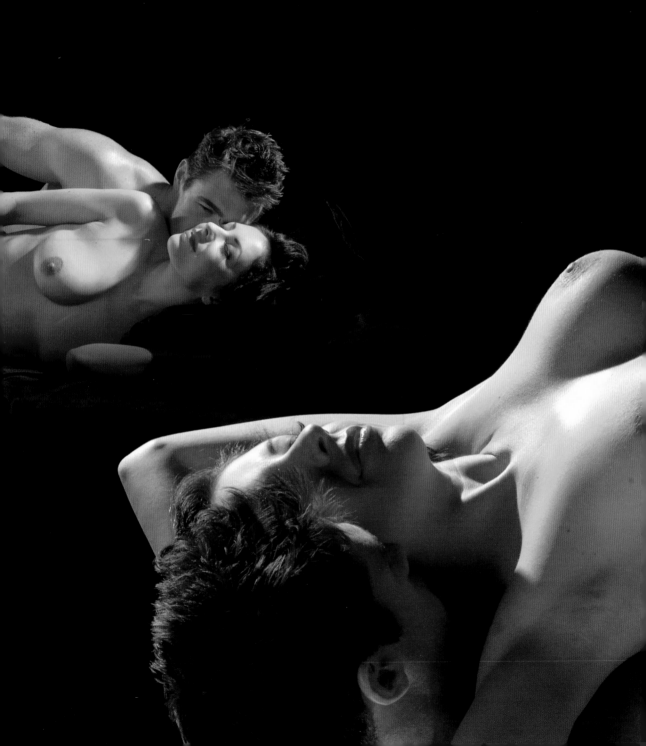

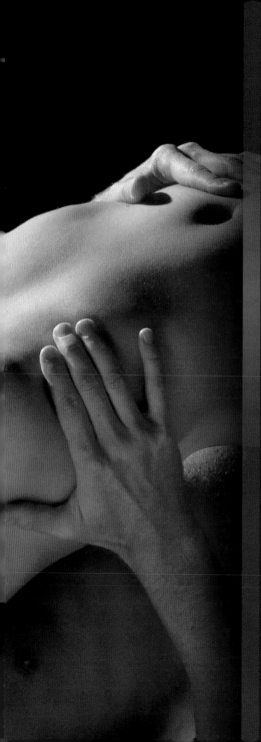

Post-Coital Cuddles

7

✳ ✳ ✳

You've just read through a lot of information on the art of cunnilingus, probably more than you've ever read or heard on this subject. People tend not to like to talk about sex in a fun AND informative way, so good for you for taking the time to learn more about oral sex on a vulva. Whether you read the book straight through or flipped through to the pictures that interested you or the sections that grabbed your attention, you're ahead of the pack in knowing more about vulvar anatomy, communication skills, sex toys, lube and safe sex, and of course, steamy positions than the average lover.

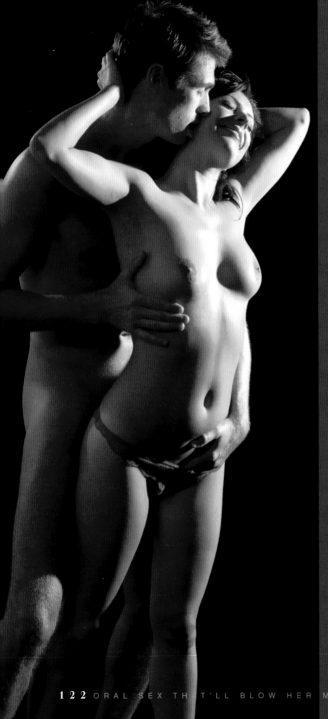

Use this knowledge how you choose; if you're currently partnered, surprise your lover with newer and spicier adventures in the boudoir. If you're sleeping around, show off your skill set with anyone you deem worthy of sharing cunnilingus. I suggest not using every single trick, tip, and technique in one go. Rather, spread them out, and the two of you can explore them all and then pick out your absolute favorites, save the ones that are pretty good for future sexy times, and leave the ones that just got a "meh" in the dust. Please don't hurt yourself or your partner in trying new things . . . and if you do, remember, there's should be no shame in telling the doctor that you hurt yourself while on a sexual adventure. If you'd prefer not to mention how you got hurt, that's fine too—just make sure you and your partner get the medical care you need.

It's incredibly important to remember a few things. First of all, there are no such things as sex experts. We're constantly learning about sex and bodies as a whole, as well as learning the individual ins and outs, wants and needs, pleasure zones, and more for each individual person. Don't beat yourself up if something you try doesn't quite work; just smile, laugh about it, and move on to something else fun that you both enjoy, or try out something else new and different. The other thing to remember is that there's no holy grail or magic formula for cunnilingus, as much as many of us wish there were. If you want to be amazing at giving fabulous cunnilingus, you need to take what your particular partner likes into consideration, communicate with them, listen to their feedback and assimilate it into your skill set, and remember that practice can lead to pleasure. The more you experiment and get to know their body, mind, and desires, the better the sex will be for the both of you.

So with all of this in mind, go forth into the world and share your exciting carnal knowledge with the one (or ones) whom you love and desire. Explore the world of sexuality, experiment with new ideas and positions, and remember the importance of having this trifecta: communication, lubrication, and laughter. With these three items and the knowledge from this book on your side, you're sure to have a fun and fabulous time whenever you decide to dine out at the Y!

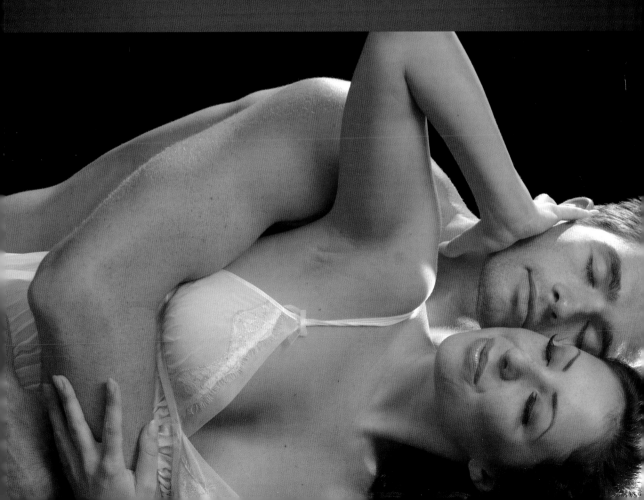

About the Author

Shanna Katz, M.Ed, ACS, is a queer, kinky, disabled, feisty, femme, board-certified sexologist, sexuality educator, and professional pervert. From topics like cunnilingus and consensual nonmonogamy to communication skills and fantasies, she talks, writes, and teaches about the huge spectrum of sexuality, both from personal and professional perspectives. She's using her master's of sexuality education to provide accessible, open-source sex education to people around the country. For more information, please visit her sexuality education site, www.ShannaKatz.com.